NEPHROLOGY

MEDICAL EXAMINATION REVIEW
VOLUME 34

NEPHROLOGY

THIRD EDITION

1001 MULTIPLE CHOICE QUESTIONS AND REFERENCED EXPLANATORY ANSWERS

Edited by

Earl C. Smith, M.D.

George Dunea, M.D., F.R.C.P.

Veerasamy K.G. Pillay, M.D., M.B., Ch.B., F.R.C.P.

MEDICAL EXAMINATION PUBLISHING CO., INC.
an Excerpta Medica company

Main entry under title:

Medical examination review.

Vol. 34 published in New Hyde Park, N. Y.
Includes various editions of some volumes.
Includes bibliographical references.
1. Medicine—Examinations, questions, etc.
RC58. M4 610'. 76 61-66847
ISBN 0-87488-464-0

an Excerpta Medica company
3003 New Hyde Park Road
New Hyde Park, NY

Printed in the United States of America

Contents

About the Editors

EARL C. SMITH, M. D., Associate Professor of Medicine, Rush Medical College; Chief, Division of Nephrology, Mount Sinai Hospital Medical Center

GEORGE DUNEA, M. D., F. R. C. P., Professor of Medicine, University of Health Sciences/The Chicago Medical School; Director, Division of Nephrology-Hypertension, Cook County Hospital

VEERASAMY K. G. PILLAY, M. D., M. B., Ch. D., F. R. C. P., Professor of Medicine, University of Illinois College of Medicine at Chicago; Associate Chief of Staff for Education, Veterans Administration Westside Hospital

Chicago, Illinois

Contributors

MOHAMMAD M. AHMED, M. D., Assistant Professor of Medicine, Rush Medical College; Attending Physician, Division of Nephrology, Mount Sinai Hospital Medical Center

ASAD A. BAKIR, M. D., Director, Dialysis Unit at Cook County Hospital; Assistant Professor of Medicine, University of Health Sciences/Chicago Medical School

NADINE BAZILINSKI, M. D., Attending Nephrologist, Cook County Hospital

SURESH HATHIWALA, M. D., Attending Nephrologist, Cook County Hospital

Chicago, Illinois

Preface

Continuing advances in medical knowledge during the 8 years since the publication of the first edition have produced an even greater demand for study material to supplement standard books and journals. The third edition, revised and fully updated, seeks to meet this need. To accomplish this we have added a considerable amount of new material, to the extent that some sections have been completely recast. Whenever possible the new concepts in hypertension, renal physiology, or clinical medicine have been incorporated so as to maintain an even balance between basic sciences and practical diagnostic or therapeutic applications.

As in former editions, the material is arranged in the question and answer format. This is designed to simulate as closely as possible actual examination conditions. It should also help to promote active study habits, encouraging the student of nephrology to think about a given problem before reading the explanatory answer.

We have reduced the number of reference books to facilitate easier access to the original texts, but thought it advisable to retain the two review series to allow the presentation of new information that has not yet found its way into standard textbooks. As in the past, we have included for each question a brief explanatory answer, generally based on the textbook indicated by the reference. We suggest that the reader review each section sequentially, following up the answer with further reading of the reference textbook. We would be surprised, indeed, if some questions did not turn out to be controversial — some disagreement is to be expected in a constantly changing discipline. Less excusable, but perhaps unavoidable, is the presence of an occasional error, which even the most assiduous reviewing may fail to eradicate. But we hope that the reader will find the text sound and, if it does no more than stimulate his interest, we shall have accomplished our purpose.

notice

1. PHYSIOLOGY

DIRECTIONS: Each of the questions or incomplete statements below is followed by a list of suggested answers or completions. Select the one that is best in each case.

---

1. Which of the following is true about the juxtamedullary nephrons ?
   A. Their loops of Henle extend deep into the medulla
   B. Their glomeruli are placed most superficially in the cortex
   C. Their loops of Henle are very short
   D. They constitute 85% of all nephrons
   E. They are least effective in reabsorbing sodium
   REF. 8, p. 7

2. A 46-year-old man with advanced alcoholic liver disease has gross ascites, mild peripheral edema, and blood pressure of 90/65 mmHg. Which of the following methods would be appropriate to increase his plasma volume ?
   A. Infusion of physiologic saline
   B. Infusion of 5% dextrose in water
   C. Infusion of water
   D. Infusion of high molecular weight dextran
   E. Infusion of Ringer's lactate
   REF. 10, p. 110

3. In lactic acidosis
   A. the serum phosphate level is usually low
   B. hypercapnia, polyuria, and polydypsia are usually present but respiratory alkalosis is rare
   C. a lactate/pyruvate ratio greater than 30 indicates adequate tissue oxygenation
   D. the onset is rarely sudden, and dehydration is usually more severe than with ketoacidosis
   E. alanine, proline, and valine are elevated in the plasma but do not significantly increase the anion gap
   REF. 12(2), pp. 75-79

4. During acute acidosis, tissue glutamine decreases in all nephron segments; however, in prolonged acidosis, phosphate-dependent glutaminase is increased only in the proximal convoluted tubule. NH_3 production during acidosis is
   A. enhanced in the proximal convoluted tubule only
   B. enhanced in all nephron segments
   C. enhanced in the distal segment only
   D. decreased in all nephron segments
   E. decreased in the proximal convoluted tubule only
   REF. 10, p. 180

5. Dopamine causes renal vasoconstriction with very high doses and renal vasodilation with low doses. Renal vasodilatation with this agent is reversed by
   A. beta-adrenergic blockade
   B. prior treatment with atropine
   C. phenothiazines
   D. prior treatment with reserpine
   E. none of the above
   REF. 10, p. 278

6. Which of the following statements about alcoholic ketoacidosis is FALSE?
   A. The NADH/NAD ratio is increased
   B. The acetoacetate/beta-hydroxybutyrate ratio is increased
   C. Glucose is the most effective treatment and addition of either insulin or bicarbonate is usually unnecessary
   D. Hyperphosphatemia is common on admission
   E. Alcohol levels are usually normal on admission
   REF. 8, p. 131

7. When fat catabolism occurs and ketosis develops, the major urinary abnormality is
   A. increased excretion of uric acid
   B. mainly excretion of beta-hydroxybutyrate
   C. mainly excretion of acetone
   D. mainly excretion of acetoacetate
   REF. 5, p. 1345

8. Phosphoenolpyruvate carboxykinase is the enzyme involved in the regulation of renal gluconeogenesis. Its activity is increased during acidosis despite the concurrent use of actinomycin D. Activation of this enzyme by acidosis could be the result of
   A. synthesis of new enzyme protein
   B. conversion of the inactive enzyme to the active form
   C. increase in the decay of enzyme activity
   D. gluconeogenesis
   E. new peptide formation
   REF. 10, p. 211

9. The pathogenesis of hypernatremia from tube feeding is
   A. increased proximal tubule sodium absorption
   B. osmotic diuresis
   C. depressed antidiuretic hormone (ADH) secretion
   D. increased aldosterone secretion
   E. increased glomerular filtration
   REF. 5, p. 1444

10. Which of the following is most important in hyperalimentation solution?
   A. D-amino acids
   B. Glucose
   C. Water
   D. Potassium
   E. Multiple vitamins
   REF. 5, p. 416

11. Hyperthyroidism is associated with
   A. normal filtration fraction
   B. decreased glomerular filtration
   C. decreased renal plasma flow
   D. decreased Tm glucose
   E. decreased total body water
   REF. 5, p. 1307

12. Heat acclimatization should be done by
   A. daily increases in exercise time by 10 minutes
   B. slow daily increases in frequency of exercise for 1 month
   C. 100 minutes daily exercise for 10 days
   D. 120 minutes twice daily exercise for 5 days
   E. none of the above
   REF. 5, p. 1525

13. Exposure to heat results in all of the following EXCEPT
    A. decreased glomerular filtration
    B. increased filtration fraction
    C. inhibition of antidiuretic hormone
    D. reduced urinary sodium
    E. reduced body potassium
    REF. 5, p. 1524

14. Findings in heat stroke include all but which of the following?
    A. Hyperuricemia
    B. Hyperkalemia
    C. Hypokalemia
    D. Disproportionately high creatinine to urea blood levels
    E. Oliguria
    REF. 5, p. 1547

15. Cooling of a cell results in
    A. outward movement of sodium
    B. inward movement of potassium
    C. swelling of the cell
    D. no change in chloride transport
    E. increased transmembrane potential difference
    REF. 5, p. 26

16. Hypothyroidism is associated with all of the following EXCEPT
    A. diminished glomerular filtration
    B. intact concentrating ability
    C. inability to excrete a water load
    D. increased total body sodium
    E. decreased total body potassium
    REF. 5, p. 1306

17. Which of the following substances is most actively secreted in the colon?
    A. Sodium
    B. Potassium
    C. Chloride
    D. Bicarbonate
    E. Magnesium
    REF. 5, p. 1273

18. In a stressful situation renal blood flow
   A. decreases more than glomerular filtration rate
   B. decreases to the same extent as glomerular filtration rate
   C. decreases less than glomerular filtration rate
   D. increases while glomerular filtration rate decreases
   E. decreases while glomerular filtration rate increases
   REF. 10, p. 302

19. The distribution of blood flow within the kidney may be determined by all EXCEPT
   A. fractional uptake of radioactive potassium by tissues
   B. fractional uptake of radioactive rubidium by tissues
   C. dye-dilution curve with Evans blue
   D. radioactive krypton
   E. inulin
   REF. 10, p. 265

20. In a 90-year-old man without renal disease, the glomerular filtration rate and renal blood flow are
   A. normal
   B. 90% of normal
   C. 75% of normal
   D. 50% of normal
   E. 25% of normal
   REF. 7, p. 46

21. In moderate doses all of the following reduce renal blood flow EXCEPT
   A. epinephrine
   B. norepinephrine
   C. vasopressin
   D. renin
   E. angiotensin
   REF. 10, p. 277

22. Factors causing diminished renal blood flow include all of the following EXCEPT
   A. upright posture
   B. cold
   C. exercise
   D. pain
   E. high output cardiac failure
   REF. 10, p. 274

23. The glomerular basement membrane (GBM) contains all of the following carbohydrates EXCEPT
    A. glucose
    B. galactose
    C. fucose
    D. mannose
    E. fructose
    REF. 3, p. 18

24. Which of the following substances is concentrated in the endothelial side of the basement membrane?
    A. Horseradish peroxidase
    B. Catalase
    C. Ferritin
    D. Myloperoxidase
    E. None of the above
    REF. 3, p. 638

25. The primary filtration barrier to albumin is in the region of the
    A. lamina densa
    B. endothelium
    C. mesangial cells
    D. podocytes
    E. slit pore
    REF. 7, p. 14

26. The filtration fraction is increased in
    A. acute glomerulonephritis
    B. chronic glomerulonephritis
    C. nephrosclerosis
    D. subacute glomerulonephritis
    E. tubular necrosis
    REF. 10, p. 1355

27. Disposal of glomerular filtration residues is a function of
    A. mesangial cells
    B. epithelial cells
    C. endothelial cells
    D. basement membrane
    E. podocytes
    REF. 7, p. 13

28. Proteinuria may be induced in normal subjects by
    A. exercise
    B. salt depletion
    C. surgery
    D. injection of epinephrine
    E. all of the above
    REF. 7, p. 66

29. The tubular lumen of the ascending limb of the loop of Henle is
    A. electrically negative
    B. made positive with oubain
    C. made positive with sulfate
    D. made positive with urea
    E. electrically positive
    REF. 10, p. 344

30. The descending limb of the loop of Henle is most permeable to
    A. sodium
    B. chloride
    C. urea
    D. water
    E. bicarbonate
    REF. 10, p. 342

31. The site of final concentration of urine is the
    A. ascending limb of the loop of Henle
    B. distal tubule
    C. collecting duct
    D. distal tubule and ascending limb of the loop of Henle
    E. proximal and distal tubules
    REF. 7, p. 58

32. In the thick ascending limb of the Henle loop, the transepithelial voltage is positive in the lumen, thus
    A. sodium chloride is actively transported out of the lumen
    B. chloride is actively transported out of the lumen
    C. bicarbonate is actively transported out of the lumen
    D. hydrogen is actively transported out of the lumen
    E. water is actively transported out of the lumen
    REF. 10, p. 344

33. With regard to the tubular fluid at the tip of the loop of Henle
    A. the tubular fluid is concentrated mainly by the osmotic removal of sodium
    B. equilibration occurs mainly by osmotic addition of water to tubular fluid
    C. equilibration with interstitium is nearly complete
    D. tubular urea concentration exceeds that of the interstitium
    E. interstitial sodium concentration exceeds that of the tubular fluid

    REF. 6, p. 417

34. Match the appropriate tonicity with each region of the nephron.
    1. Isotonic
    2. Hypotonic
    3. Hypertonic

    A. Bowman space
    B. Proximal convoluted tubule
    C. Descending loop of Henle
    D. Thin limb of Henle

    REF. 7, p. 56

35. The proximal tubular fluid is
    A. hyperosmotic in diabetes insipidus
    B. isosmotic in diabetes insipidus
    C. hyposmotic with mannitol diuresis
    D. hyperosmotic with urea diuresis
    E. hyposmotic with saline diuresis

    REF. 10, p. 496

36. Which factor has the most significant effect on sodium reabsorption in the proximal tubule?
    A. Aldosterone
    B. Acute change of extracellular fluid volume
    C. Glomerular filtration rate
    D. Change of renal blood flow
    E. Changes of the concentration of blood phosphate

    REF. 2, p. 1601

37. Tubular secretion occurs with all of the following substances EXCEPT
    A. ammonia
    B. hydrogen ions
    C. potassium
    D. phosphate
    E. uric acid
    REF. 13, p. 767

38. Which of the following drugs are excreted in larger amounts in an acid urine?
    A. Acetazolamide
    B. Phenobarbital
    C. Nitrofurantoin
    D. Sulfadimidine
    E. Amphetamine
    REF. 10, p. 2662

39. The hippurate mechanism of proximal tubular secretion is involved in the transport of all of the following EXCEPT
    A. aminohippuric acid (PAH)
    B. penicillin
    C. benzathiadiazines
    D. hexamethonium
    E. phenylbutazone
    REF. 13, p. 624

40. Probenecid blocks the secretion of
    A. potassium
    B. hydrogen
    C. gentamicin
    D. EDTA
    E. penicillin
    REF. 10, p. 1035

41. Citrate excretion decreases during acidosis and during potassium depletion but increases following the administration of alkali. From this it can be concluded that the major factor regulating citrate excretion rate is
    A. extracellular fluid acidosis
    B. intracellular fluid alkalosis
    C. extracellular fluid alkalosis
    D. intracellular fluid acidosis
    E. alkaline urine
    REF. 10, p. 199

42. With reference to the renal excretion of PAH, which of the following statements is FALSE?
   A. The amount excreted is the sum of glomerular filtration and tubular secretion
   B. At low plasma levels, the amount secreted exceeds considerably the amount filtered at the glomerulus
   C. Tm PAH is defined as the value beyond which excretion takes place only by secretion
   D. The splay in the titration curve for PAH is due to heterogeneity of the nephrons' perfusion/transport capacity ratio
   E. At plasma PAH levels of about 2 mg/100 ml, roughly 90% of the PAH brought to the kidney is removed during one passage

   REF. 7, p. 55

43. Increasing osmotic load to the kidney while under maximal ADH stimulation results in
   A. increased urine flow
   B. increased urine concentration
   C. no change in urine concentration
   D. increased medullary osmolality
   E. decreased solute output

   REF. 7, p. 1485

44. The fluid in the early distal convoluted tubule is hypotonic to plasma because of
   A. antidiuretic hormone
   B. sodium and chloride reabsorption at the diluting sites
   C. equilibration with the interstitium
   D. dissipation of the medullary interstitial gradient
   E. aldosterone secretion

   REF. 7, p. 1480

45. With regard to nonionic diffusion, which of the following statements is true?
   A. Water-soluble substances can pass with ease through membrane pores, and therefore permeate easily across cells
   B. Lipid-soluble substances must pass through the whole thickness of the membrane, and therefore permeate cells with difficulty
   C. Weak bases diffuse out of the tubular lumen more rapidly as the pH decreases
   D. Weak acids diffuse out of the tubular lumen more rapidly as the pH decreases
   E. The urinary excretion of weak basis is greatest when the urine is alkalinized

   REF. 7(2nd ed.), p. 77

46. With regard to the effect of increasing peritubular colloid osmotic pressure on sodium reabsorption
    A. passive reabsorption decreases dramatically
    B. active reabsorption decreases dramatically
    C. active reabsorption increases but passive reabsorption decreases
    D. passive reabsorption increases more than active reabsorption
    E. active reabsorption increases more than passive reabsorption
    REF. 7, p. 1515

47. With regard to the cellular action of vasopressin, which of the following apply?
    A. Vasopressin is bound to receptors on the luminal surface of tubule
    B. Vasopressin is bound to receptors on the basolateral surface of tubule
    C. After attachment of vasopressin to receptors phosphodiesterase is activated
    D. Binding of vasopressin to receptor is irreversible
    E. Receptor occupance is high during diuresis
    REF. 10, p. 793

48. Regarding the relationship of urinary volume, plasma osmolality (P_{osm}), osmolar clearance (C_{osm}), and free water clearance ($C\ H_2O$), which of the following statements is true?
    A. When U_{osm} equals P_{osm}, then $C\ H_2O$ is negative
    B. As C_{osm} and urine volume increase, $C\ H_2O$ decreases
    C. When U_{osm} is greater than P_{osm} then $C\ H_2O$ becomes positive
    D. When $C\ H_2O$ is negative, then C_{osm} is greater than urinary volume
    E. When U_{osm} is less than P_{osm}, then $C\ H_2O$ equals urinary volume
    REF. 7, p. 1486

49. Which of the following does NOT increase the difference between the measured and calculated osmolality by more than 10 mOsm/kg H_2O?
    A. Urea
    B. Mannitol
    C. Methanol
    D. Ethanol
    E. Ethylene glycol
    REF. 12(1), pp. 1, 2

50. Diabetes insipidus rather than compulsive polydypsia is more likely if
   A. plasma osmolality is 260 mOsm/kg water
   B. the patient is a woman with a history of psychiatric disorder
   C. there is a considerable variation in water intake
   D. the onset of the disorder is sudden
   E. the polyuria responds to fluid restriction
   REF. 2, p. 610

51. Regarding diabetes insipidus, which of the following statements is true?
   A. The condition is frequently mistaken for compulsive polydypsia, but treatment is the same
   B. Most patients have an underlying defect in the area striata
   C. Water restriction will usually abolish the polyuria
   D. Thiazide diuretics are effective because they cause hypokalemia
   E. Thiazide diuretics are effective because they contract the extracellular volume
   REF. 2, p. 606

52. Hypercalcemia causes polyuria by inhibiting
   A. binding of vasopressin to its receptors
   B. cyclic AMP action
   C. phosphodiesterase
   D. cyclic AMP destruction
   E. sodium transport
   REF. 10, p. 794

53. Which of the following does NOT cause nephrogenic diabetes insipidus?
   A. Demeclocycline
   B. Pyelonephritis
   C. Lithium
   D. Obstructive uropathy
   E. Penicillin
   REF. 10, p. 800

54. Total body water is best measured by
   A. Evans blue
   B. radioiodinated human serum albumin
   C. deuterium oxide
   D. radioactive phosphorus
   E. radioactive chromium
   REF. 10, p. 89

55. Sodium and water transport is increased in the toad bladder by all of the following EXCEPT
    A. cyclic AMP
    B. phosphodiesterase
    C. ADH
    D. theophylline
    E. decreased acidity of serosal fluid
    REF. 7, p. 1476

56. The lowest percent of body water in relation to weight is found in
    A. an obese person
    B. a lean person
    C. a tall person
    D. an infant
    E. a muscular person
    REF. 7, p. 1507

57. The osmolality of urine of man
    A. reaches only 100 m0sm/kg in water diuresis
    B. reaches less than 30 m0sm/kg in water diuresis
    C. reaches only 900 m0sm/kg in hydropenia
    D. is isosmolal to plasma with hydropenia
    E. is isosmolal to plasma with water diuresis
    REF. 7, p. 1486

58. Both sodium and calcium excretion are increased with
    A. acute desoxycorticosterone administration
    B. chronic desoxycorticosterone administration
    C. parathormone administration
    D. chronic chlorothiazide therapy
    E. acute furosemide ingestion
    REF. 7, pp. 1409-1415

59. Which is a sensitive indicator of water conservation at low urine flow?
    A. Rate of urine flow
    B. Urine/plasma (U/P) creatinine ratio
    C. Urinary creatinine concentration
    D. Serum creatinine
    E. Urinary urea concentration
    REF. 7, p. 1486

60. If the serum sodium concentration increases by 25%, which of the following has occurred?
A. Total body water has decreased by 25%
B. Total body water has decreased by 50%
C. Extracellular water has decreased by 25%
D. Extracellular water has decreased by 50%
E. None of the above
REF. 5, p. 1450

61. Hypernatremia can result in all of the following EXCEPT
A. myoclonis
B. diminished deep tendon reflexes
C. seizures
D. mental confusion
E. increased cerebrospinal fluid pressure
REF. 5, p. 502

62. Most of the sodium in the body is located in the
A. plasma
B. interstitial fluid
C. intracellular fluid
D. bone
E. muscle cells
REF. 5, p. 1065

63. Extracellular sodium is what percent of the total body sodium?
A. 95%
B. 66%
C. 50%
D. 33%
E. 25%
REF. 5, p. 13

64. Which of the following is the poorest stimulus for natriuresis?
A. Blood
B. Plasma
C. Saline
D. Albumin
E. Ringer's solution
REF. 5, p. 250

65. All of the following substances are natriuretic EXCEPT
    A. 17 hydroxprogesterone
    B. spironolactone
    C. progesterone
    D. angiotensin II
    E. estrogens
    REF. 5, p. 1304

66. Which of the following substances have their excretion rate determined only by plasma concentration ?
    A. Sodium
    B. Calcium
    C. Phosphate
    D. Creatinine
    E. Uric acid
    REF. 5, p. 236

67. In the hydropenic state, permeability to water is lowest in the
    A. proximal tubule
    B. descending limb of the loop of Henle
    C. ascending limb of the loop of Henle
    D. cortical segment of the collecting duct
    E. medullary segment of the collecting duct
    REF. 7, p. 1479

68. Antidiuresis unrelated to change in osmolality of body fluids is induced by all of the following EXCEPT
    A. infusion of iso-oncotic albumin
    B. assumption of erect posture
    C. positive-pressure breathing
    D. hemorrhage
    E. venous tourniquets to the lower limbs
    REF. 10, p. 778

69. Which of the following inhibits ADH release ?
    A. Emotional stress
    B. Isoproterenol
    C. Extracellular volume contraction
    D. Acetylcholine
    E. Phenytoin (Dilantin)
    REF. 5, p. 566

70. Which of the following statements about antidiuretic hormone is true?
    A. It decreases the permeability of the collecting duct to urea
    B. It inhibits sodium transport
    C. It stimulates sodium transport
    D. It promotes passive movement of sodium
    E. It promotes active water transport
    REF. 6, p. 792

71. Antidiuretic hormone
    A. catalyzes the conversion of 3'5 adenosine monophosphate (cyclic AMP) to adenosine triphosphate (ATP)
    B. increases tubular permeability by acting at the basal (antiluminal) surface of the cell
    C. retards sodium transport by inhibiting phosphodiesterase
    D. causes phosphodiesterase to activate a protein kinase
    E. activates membrane-bound adenylcyclase at the blood surface
    REF. 6, p. 792

72. With regard to ADH, which of the following statements is true?
    A. It is a decapeptide
    B. In the pig, arginine replaces lysine
    C. It is synthesized by the cells of the posterior pituitary
    D. It migrates via the supraoptic-hypophyseal tract to the hypothalamus
    E. Its release is regulated by vesicular cells in the supraoptic nucleus
    REF. 7, p. 1476

73. Which of the following do NOT stimulate ADH release?
    A. Hypertonic saline infusion
    B. Urea infusion
    C. Water deprivation
    D. Hemorrhage
    E. Positive-pressure breathing
    REF. 5, p. 566

74. Which of the following drugs is antidiuretic?
    A. Morphine
    B. Propoxyphene
    C. Colchicine
    D. Lithium
    E. Alcohol
    REF. 12, (1), p. 12

75. Which of the following drugs inhibit antidiuretic hormone secretion?
A. Morphine
B. Barbiturates
C. Nicotine
D. Alcohol
E. Histamine
REF. 8, p. 49

76. The secretion of ADH is "appropriate" to maintain effective plasma volume in all of the following EXCEPT
A. cirrhosis of the liver
B. renal vein thrombosis
C. congestive heart failure
D. gastrointestinal fluid losses
E. bronchogenic carcinoma
REF. 12(1), pp. 13, 154-163

77. Which of the following antidiuretic drugs may act directly on the kidney?
A. Clofibrate
B. Nicotine
C. Morphine
D. Chlorpropamide
E. Carbamazepine
REF. 12(1), p. 12

78. Which of the following statements is FALSE?
A. High calcium concentrations antagonize the action of antidiuretic hormone probably by inhibiting the interaction between hormone and receptors, and by inhibiting adenylate cyclase activation
B. Prostaglandin E antagonizes the action of vasopressin by inhibiting adenylate cyclase
C. Aldosterone antagonizes the effects of vasopressin
D. Beta-adrenergic agents produce antidiuresis probably by increasing adenylate cyclase activity
E. Alpha-adrenergic agents exert a diuretic effect probably by inhibiting adenylate cyclase
REF. 6, pp. 806-807

79. Which of the following drugs causes diabetes insipidus?
A. Demeclocycline
B. Chlorpropamide
C. Cyclophosphamide
D. Clofibrate
E. Carbamazepine
REF. 10, p. 800

80. Which of the following drugs is antidiuretic?
    A. Diphenylhydantoin
    B. Isoproterenol
    C. Colchicine
    D. Epinephrine
    E. Alcohol
    REF. 12(1), p. 12

81. Effective plasma volume is normal or increased in all but which of the following causes of hyponatremia?
    A. Beer potomania
    B. Inappropriate antidiuretic hormone secretion
    C. Addison's disease
    D. Compulsive polydipsia
    E. Clofibrate administration
    REF. 8, p. 44

82. Which of the following may play a role in the hyponatremia of hypothyroidism?
    A. Increased delivery of filtrate to the diluting sites
    B. An alcohol-like effect of thyroxin deficiency
    C. Increased cortisol secretion
    D. Increased antidiuretic hormone secretion
    E. Release of water and sodium from myxomatous tissue
    REF. 8, p. 48

83. Hyponatremia in congestive heart failure is NOT due to which of the following?
    A. Increased antidiuretic hormone secretion
    B. Decreased filtrate delivery to the distal tubules
    C. Increased effective plasma volume
    D. Decreased cardiac output
    E. Increased proximal sodium reabsorption
    REF. 8, p. 44

84. Which of the following changes is most likely in the syndrome of inappropriate ADH secretion?
    A. Elevated plasma urea
    B. Decreased effective plasma volume
    C. Reduced urinary sodium excretion
    D. Decreased proximal tubular sodium reabsorption
    E. Abnormal adrenal function
    REF. 1, p. 477

85. Inappropriate antidiuretic hormone secretion is seen with all of the following EXCEPT
   A. head trauma
   B. cavernous sinus thrombosis
   C. lithium intoxication
   D. porphyria
   E. meningitis
   REF. 8, p. 50

86. Which of the following patients is LEAST likely to present with hyponatremia?
   A. An epileptic who stops her phenytoin and not only continues her carbamazepine but on developing convulsions increases the dosage
   B. A diabetic with heart failure treated with chlorpropamide and hydrochlorothiazide
   C. A diabetic with heart failure treated with phenytoin and acetohexamide
   D. A man with carcinoma of the lung treated with morphine, barbiturates, and cyclophosphamide
   E. A woman with leukemia receiving vincristine and acetaminophen
   REF. 8, pp. 31, 49

87. Free water clearance
   A. is positive when the urine is hypertonic
   B. is increased by furosemide
   C. in severe water diuresis may reach a maximum of 3 ml/min
   D. is decreased by acetozolamide administration
   E. in the absence of ADH, represents sodium transport at diluting sites
   REF. 12(1), pp. 585, 673

88. Regarding the clinical criteria for the syndrome of inappropriate antidiuretic hormone (SIADH), which of the following does NOT apply?
   A. Urinary sodium excretion is low in relation to serum sodium
   B. Low serum osmolality
   C. Urine osmolality is usually higher than serum osmolality
   D. Hyponatremia
   E. Serum osmolality returns to normal with water restriction
   REF. 10, p. 820

89. All of the following substances injected into a carotid artery will not stimulate ADH release EXCEPT
A. mannitol
B. glucose
C. sodium
D. urea
E. dextran
REF. 5, p. 567

90. Increased Na excretion from the proximal tubule is produced in all of the following experimental conditions EXCEPT
A. rise in peritubular pressure
B. fall in plasma protein osmotic pressure
C. increased circulating blood volume
D. by infusion of "unknown hormone" from a volume-expanded animal
E. renal artery constriction
REF. 13, p. 107

91. Evidence that Na transport is an active process may come from which of the following?
A. Under normal conditions the tubular fluid in the proximal tubule remains isosmotic to plasma
B. Under normal conditions the tubular fluid is hypertonic to plasma
C. There is a linear relationship between renal oxygen consumption and Na reabsorption
D. There is a steep gradient of Na ion concentration between the tubular fluid and the peritubular fluid under normal circumstances
E. None of the above
REF. 10, p. 146

92. Hypernatremia in the presence of uncontrolled diabetes mellitus suggests
A. salt overload
B. water depletion
C. hyperlipemia
D. increased tubular Na resorption
E. ketoacidosis
REF. 5, p. 1341

93. The edema associated with refeeding after a fast is probably due to
   A. hypoalbuminemia
   B. salt retention
   C. increased vascular permeability
   D. increased protein synthesis
   E. none of the above
   REF. 5, p. 1498

94. In the presence of severe hyperlipidemia and a normal amount of sodium in the plasma water, the concentration of sodium in total plasma will appear to be
   A. normal
   B. increased
   C. decreased
   D. unpredictable
   E. dependent on turbidity
   REF. 5, p. 12

95. Patients with idiopathic edema who are given a salt load usually have
   A. diminished urinary sodium excretion
   B. no change in urinary sodium excretion
   C. increased sodium excretion in urine
   D. no predictable pattern
   E. acute pulmonary edema
   REF. 5, p. 537

96. A patient has a serum sodium level of 170 mEq/L and a urine sodium level of 10 mEq/L. The most likely diagnosis is
   A. infusion of hypertonic saline
   B. water deprivation
   C. tube feeding
   D. diabetes insipidus
   E. diuretic abuse
   REF. 5, p. 607

97. In dehydration, infusion of hypertonic saline will result in
   A. decrease in urinary output
   B. increase in urine osmolality
   C. fall in concentration of excreted substances in urine
   D. decrease in serum osmolality
   E. no change in urine and serum osmolality
   REF. 10, p. 789

98. A low serum potassium is LEAST serious in which of the following?
   A. Digitalis administration
   B. Cirrhosis
   C. Metabolic alkalosis
   D. Respiratory acidosis
   E. Metabolic acidosis
   REF. 8, p. 142

99. Potassium reabsorption
   A. is largely passive
   B. depends mainly on dietary potassium
   C. takes place mainly in the distal nephron
   D. is modulated by aldosterone
   E. may occur in the collecting duct
   REF. 7, p. 1588

100. Regarding potassium excretion, which of the following statements is FALSE?
   A. It occurs mainly in the distal tubule and is actively transported
   B. It depends on a 1:1 exchange with sodium and varies inversely with the hydrogen ion
   C. Its rate of secretion is proportional to the intracellular potassium pool
   D. Diffusion down a favorable electrochemical gradient occurs because the lumen is electronegative and the potassium concentration lower
   E. In the collecting duct it may be effected by an ATPase mediated sodium-potassium exchange mechanism
   REF. 2, p. 1605

101. Distal tubular potassium secretion is reduced by
   A. increased proximal sodium reabsorption
   B. potassium loading
   C. aldosterone
   D. respiratory acidosis
   E. metabolic acidosis
   REF. 12(2), pp. 20-25

102. The most important site for regulation of potassium excretion is
   A. proximal convoluted tubule
   B. ascending loop of Henle
   C. distal convoluted tubule
   D. collecting duct
   E. descending limb of Henle
   REF. 2, p. 1605

103. Hypokalemia may cause all but which of the following?
A. Polyuria and polydipsia
B. Hyperphosphatemia
C. Increased ammonia production
D. Tetany
E. Edema and sodium retention
REF. 2, p. 1659

104. Potassium deficiency causes
A. increased reabsorption of sodium by the proximal tubule
B. natriuresis
C. increased total body sodium
D. increased aldosterone level
E. decreased renin level
REF. 7, p. 1594

105. Which of the following is more related to human K depletion?
A. Vacuoles in the cortical tubules
B. Hyperplasia of the collecting duct
C. Vacuoles in the glomeruli
D. Vacuoles in the collecting duct
E. Vacuoles in the interstitium
REF. 2, p. 1659

106. Which of the following is most commonly found in K depletion?
A. Loss of urine concentration ability
B. Reduction in glomerular filtration rate (GFR)
C. Loss of urinary diluting capacity
D. Impairment of free water clearance
E. Reduction in PAH clearance
REF. 2, p. 1659

107. All of the following are caused by K depletion EXCEPT
A. reduction of aldosterone secretion
B. augmented ammonia production
C. increased renin level
D. impairment of chloride reabsorption
E. hypermagnesemia
REF. 7, p. 1584

108. Which of the following factors leads to decreased potassium excretion?
A. Sodium chloride infusion
B. Furosemide
C. Aldosterone
D. Hypoaldosteronism
E. Alkalosis
REF. 5, p. 117

109. A 50-year-old diabetic man is admitted because of hyperkalemia. Serum creatinine is 5 mg% and urine volume is 950 ml/day. Which of the following statements is correct?
A. Renin hypersecretion is probably occurring
B. Aldosterone secretion is probably normal
C. The correct treatment is to restrict sodium intake
D. The patient is on the verge of developing anuria
E. Treatment with 9-alpha-fluorohydrocortisone may help
REF. 5, p. 903

110. Hypokalemia during the blastic phase of acute leukemia may be associated with all of the following EXCEPT
A. destruction of leukocytes and platelets
B. renal potassium wasting
C. hypouricemia and hypomagnesemia
D. hypocalcemia and lysozymuria
E. hyperreninism and isosthenuria
REF. 8, p. 208

111. Renal potassium excretion is increased by all of the following EXCEPT
A. a high urine flow rate
B. furosemide
C. hypoaldosteronism
D. metabolic alkalosis
E. sodium sulfate infusions
REF. 8, p. 188

112. Which of the following acute changes lowers the resting membrane potential?
A. Hyperkalemia
B. Hypokalemia
C. Hypercalcemia
D. Hypocalcemia
E. Hypokalemia plus hypercalcemia
REF. 5, p. 506

113. Which of the following ECG changes will NOT be found in a cirrhotic with chronic diarrhea who has been taking diuretics?
A. Flattened T waves
B. U waves
C. Shortened QT interval
D. ST segment depression
E. Ectopic beats
REF. 8, p. 203

114. Regarding phosphate excretion, which of the following statements is correct?
A. Less than 20% of plasma phosphorus is filtered at the glomerulus
B. The clearance of phosphate normally does not exceed 10 ml/min
C. Most of the phosphate reabsorption takes place in the proximal tubule
D. Most of the phosphate reabsorption takes place in the distal tubule
E. Phosphate secretion accounts for about half of all the excreted phosphate
REF. 10, p. 575

115. Phosphaturia occurs in
A. hypermagnesemia
B. hypomagnesemia
C. hypoparathyroidism
D. acute hypercalcemia
E. alkalosis
REF. 6, pp. 614-616

116. Which of the following hormones influences renal phosphate excretion?
A. Erythropoietin
B. Aldosterone
C. Estrogen
D. Parathormone
E. Thyroxine
REF. 10, p. 585

117. Regarding phosphate reabsorption, which of the following statements is FALSE?
   A. When the blood level of phosphate increases, a maximal capacity for tubular reabsorption is reached
   B. When the phosphate level in the blood falls, the phosphate clearance is unchanged
   C. Acidosis increases phosphorus excretion but does not lower the Tm
   D. Acetazolamide administration produces phosphaturia
   E. Glucagon administration produces phosphaturia
   REF. 6, pp. 605-614

118. Which of the following infusions may result in decreased phosphate excretion?
   A. Glucose
   B. Calcium
   C. Amino acids
   D. Acetoacetate
   E. Para-aminohippurate
   REF. 6, p. 615

119. Which of the following does NOT cause phosphaturia?
   A. Parathormone
   B. Cyclic AMP
   C. Renal vasodilatation
   D. Phlorizin
   E. Calcitonin
   REF. 6, p. 617

120. Which of the following increases phosphate reabsorption?
   A. Sodium bicarbonate
   B. Renal vasodilatation
   C. Extracellular volume expansion
   D. Dextrose-saline infusions
   E. Magnesium salts
   REF. 6, p. 616

121. Which of the following enhances tubular reabsorption of calcium?
   A. Furosemide administration
   B. Parathyroid hormone
   C. High magnesium intake
   D. Metabolic acidosis
   E. Ingestion of carbohydrate
   REF. 5, p. 349

122. Which of the following reduces the urinary excretion of calcium?
A. Sodium chloride infusion
B. Renal vasodilatation
C. Hypercalcemia
D. Furosemide
E. Phosphate loading
REF. 6, p. 570

123. Parathyroid hormone increases tubular reabsorption of calcium in the
A. proximal tubule
B. distal tubule
C. ascending limb of the loop of Henle
D. descending limb of the loop of Henle
E. collecting duct
REF. 12, p. 367

124. Metabolic acidosis increases calcium excretion by all of the following EXCEPT
A. increasing ionized calcium
B. decreasing parathormone level
C. acutely inhibiting Na^+ and Ca^+ reabsorption in parallel
D. chronically by selectively inhibiting Ca^+ reabsorption in the distal nephron
E. stimulating proximal Ca^+ secretion
REF. 10, p. 563

125. Vasodilatation and increase in perfusion pressure increase the excretion of calcium. Which of the following is NOT calciuric?
A. Acetylcholine
B. Bradykinin
C. Angiotensin
D. Angiotensin plus acetylcholine
E. Angiotensin plus aortic constriction
REF. 10, p. 564

126. Calcium reabsorption in the distal convoluted tubule
A. comprises 70% of all the filtered calcium
B. is decreased by parathormone
C. is increased by thiazide diuretics
D. parallels sodium reabsorption
E. is decreased by vitamin D
REF. 8, p. 228

127. Parathyroid hormone
A. depresses osteoclastic activity
B. decreases calcium mobilization from bone
C. increases proximal phosphate reabsorption
D. by inhibiting the formation of 1.25-dihydroxy cholecalciferol greatly enhances intestinal calcium absorption
E. depresses tubular calcium reabsorption proximally but enhances it distally
REF. 8, p. 236

128. Acute hypercalcemia may produce
A. decrease in sodium excretion
B. increase in potassium excretion
C. fall in titratable acidity
D. increase in magnesium excretion
E. tetany
REF. 10, p. 600

129. Which of the following statements about parathyroid hormone is FALSE?
A. It has a molecular weight of 9500 and consists of 84 amino acids
B. The fraction with the amino terminal has an amino acid sequence of 1 to 34, and is biologically active
C. The biologically inactive fraction has the carboxy-terminal and an amino acid sequence of 53 to 84
D. The total level of circulating parathormone is not useful in the diagnosis of hyperparathyroidism
E. Measurement of total circulating hormone levels after calcium infusion is helpful in certain clinical situations
REF. 8, p. 236

130. Which of the following is NOT hypercalciuric?
A. Administration of mannitol
B. Chronic administration of acetazolamide
C. Acute administration of thiazide diuretics
D. Chronic administration of thiazide diuretics
E. Furosemide
REF. 10, p. 567

131. Glucocorticoids can cause all of the following EXCEPT
A. increased urinary calcium excretion
B. diminished intestinal absorption of calcium
C. inhibition of bone resorption
D. increased urinary phosphate excretion
E. increased hydrogen retention
REF. 10, p. 475

132. Which of the following ions is largely reabsorbed in the distal nephron?
A. Calcium
B. Potassium
C. Phosphorus
D. Magnesium
E. Sodium
REF. 8, p. 300

133. Experimentally which of the following decreases urinary magnesium excretion?
A. Sodium loads
B. Calcium loads
C. Thiazide diuretics
D. Parathormone
E. Aldosterone
REF. 8, p. 301

134. Hypermagnesemia
A. depresses deep tendon reflexes
B. stimulates parathormone
C. increases atrioventricular conduction
D. causes vasoconstriction
E. enhances hydroxyapatite deposition
REF. 8, p. 312

135. All but which of the following are causes of hypomagnesmia?
A. Alcoholism
B. Malabsorption
C. Uremia
D. Malnutrition
E. Diuretic therapy
REF. 8, p. 308

136. What is the tubular reabsorption of bicarbonate if glomerular fitration is 100 ml/min, serum bicarbonate 30 mM/L, urine volume 60 cc/hr, and urine bicarbonate 4 mM/L?
A. 2.996 mM/min
B. 300 mM/hr
C. 2 mM/min
D. 600 mM/hr
E. None of the above
REF. 10, p. 868

137. The amount of titratable acid excretion depends mainly on
A. capacity of the buffers in the urine
B. amount of ammonium ion in the urine
C. partial pressure of O_2 in the blood
D. amount of CO_2 in the urine
E. none of the above
REF. 13, p. 588

138. The maintenance of a stable pH is the result of chemical buffering and physiologic control mechanisms. The important chemical buffers in the body include all of the following EXCEPT
A. proteins
B. phosphate
C. bicarbonate
D. sulphate
E. hemoglobin
REF. 10, p. 844

139. The major buffer for an acute acid load is
A. blood buffers
B. interstitial fluid buffers
C. cellular buffers
D. respiratory system
E. kidneys
REF. 7, p. 1549

140. The body buffer defense is poorest for
A. acute respiratory acidosis
B. acute metabolic acidosis
C. chronic respiratory alkalosis
D. chronic metabolic alkalosis
E. mixed disorders
REF. 5, p. 220

141. One millimole of carbon dioxide at standard temperature and pressure occupies
A. 2.24 ml
B. 22.4 ml
C. 224 ml
D. 224 L
E. none of the above
REF. 5, p. 4

142. The amount of sodium bicarbonate needed to increase the plasma bicarbonate concentration by the amount desired is about 50% of body weight. With regard to the treatment of metabolic acidosis, which of the following apply?
   A. In a 60 kg man 150 mEq of bicarbonate will increase plasma bicarbonate by 15 mEq/L
   B. Additional bicarbonate is needed to compensate for continued production of acid or loss of bicarbonate
   C. Complete restoration of base deficit with bicarbonate within hours is mandatory in metabolic acidosis
   D. Hyperkalemia is a complication of bicarbonate therapy in patients with metabolic acidosis
   E. The bicarbonate level is more important to follow than pH
   REF. 10, p. 885

143. Carbonic anhydrase speeds up mainly the
   A. production of carbon dioxide
   B. production of carbonic acid
   C. production of free hydrogen
   D. acidification of bicarbonate
   E. production of water
   REF. 5, p. 185

144. In hypokalemia there is
   A. extracellular acidosis
   B. intracellular alkalosis
   C. intracellular acidosis
   D. alkaline urine
   E. increased bicarbonate excretion
   REF. 7, p. 1586

145. Infusion of potassium salts results in
   A. intracellular acidosis
   B. extracellular acidosis
   C. both intracellular and extracellular acidosis
   D. acid urine
   E. extracellular alkalosis
   REF. 7, p. 1595

146. Hydrogen ion secretion is
   A. increased by extracellular fluid volume expansion
   B. enhanced by a decreased plasma PCO_2
   C. enhanced by high parathormone levels
   D. decreased by potassium depletion
   E. enhanced by aldosterone
   REF. 12 (2), pp. 12-16

147. With reference to bicarbonate reabsorption which of the following statements is FALSE?
A. Hydrogen ions are formed either by hydration of CO_2 or by a redox mechanism splitting water into hydrogen and hydroxyl ions
B. Transport of hydrogen ions is active
C. More hydrogen ion is used for bicarbonate reclamation (reabsorption) than for regeneration, but relatively more H^+ reacts with nonbicarbonate buffers as bicarbonate reabsorption nears completion
D. Within the cell carbonic anhydrase decreases the supply of H^+ to a secretory pump
E. Within the lumen carbonic anhydrase lowers the gradient against which H^+ is secreted by catalyzing carbonic acid dehydration
REF. 12(2), pp. 2-4

148. Bicarbonate reabsorption is
A. Tm-limited
B. not Tm-limited
C. not dependent on carbonic anhydrase
D. increased by acetazolamide
E. unaffected by acetazolamide
REF. 7, p. 1550

149. During alkalosis the parathormone secretion rate increases. The increase in parathormone would do all of the following EXCEPT
A. decrease bicarbonate reabsorption
B. decrease phosphate reabsorption
C. reduce renal citrate oxidation
D. stimulate carbonic anhydrase activity
E. deter cyclic AMP activity
REF. 10, p. 199

150. The increase in citrate excretion during alkalosis can be accounted for by a decrease in citrate reabsorption. Citrate reabsorption is regulated by the
A. concentration gradient for citrate between the tubule lumen and the tubule cell
B. intracellular fluid pH
C. urine pH
D. extracellular fluid pH
E. intravascular volume
REF. 10, p. 199

151. During chronic metabolic alkalosis, renal glucose utilization is four times greater than during chronic metabolic acidosis. Renal oxidation of glucose is not significantly affected by acid-base status. Metabolic alkalosis increases the conversion of glucose to
A. carbon dioxide
B. lactate
C. glycerol
D. glycogen
E. glucosamine
REF. 10, p. 204

152. Ammonia is
A. charged
B. uncharged
C. water soluble
D. penetrates cell membranes with difficulty
E. is an acid
REF. 7, p. 1552

153. Which of the following decreases ammonium excretion?
A. Potassium depletion
B. Respiratory acidosis
C. Mineral acid load
D. Ammonium chloride ingestion
E. Calcium chloride ingestion
REF. 5, p. 259

154. Which of the following is NOT measured in titratable acidity?
A. Phosphate
B. Sulfate
C. Ammonia
D. Creatinine
E. Hydrochloric acid
REF. 5, p. 258

155. Excretion of titratable acidity is increased in
A. renal tubular acidosis
B. potassium deficiency
C. hypercalcemia
D. chronic renal failure
E. none of the above
REF. 10, p. 476

156. The most common acid-base abnormality immediately following surgery is
A. respiratory acidosis
B. respiratory alkalosis
C. metabolic alkalosis
D. metabolic acidosis
E. lactic acidosis
REF. 5, p. 223

157. Rapid correction of metabolic acidosis may result in severe coma by
A. cerebrospinal fluid acidosis
B. Donnan disequilibrium
C. hypernatremia
D. hypoxia
E. respiratory alkalosis
REF. 5, p. 202

158. Metabolic acidosis with an increased anion gap is LEAST likely to occur in
A. lactic acidosis
B. uremic acidosis
C. renal tubular acidosis
D. ethylene glycol ingestion
E. diabetic ketoacidosis
REF. 8, p. 132

159. In which of the following conditions is hydrogen ion secretion likely to be greatest?
A. Chronic bronchitis with CO_2 retention
B. Alveolocapillary block
C. The administration of potassium salts
D. Acetazolamide administration
E. Hypoaldosteronism
REF. 7, pp. 1572-1574

160. An increased anion gap is compatible with which of the following?
A. Pseudomonas bacteremia treated with polymyxin B
B. Hyperalimentation
C. Rapid expansion of plasma volume
D. Paraldehyde poisoning
E. Multiple myeloma
REF. 8, p. 133

161. If a patient with acidosis has a pH of 7.2 and a HCO_3 of 10, how much bicarbonate will be required to raise his serum bicarbonate to 18 if his body weight is 60 kg?
A. 8 mEq
B. 680 mEq
C. 48 mEq
D. 240 mEq
E. 27 mEq
REF. 7, p. 1560

162. The ability to reduce the pH of the urine after the administration of 0.1 g ammonium chloride/kg body weight is LEAST likely to occur in which of the following conditions?
A. Renal tubular acidosis (distal type)
B. Hypokalemia
C. Chronic renal failure
D. Fanconi's syndrome
E. Acetazolamide administration
REF. 7, p. 1031

163. In acute respiratory acidosis the main buffering mechanism is
A. extracellular
B. cellular
C. renal
D. plasma proteins
E. bicarbonate
REF. 7, p. 1572

164. In patients with renal disease the acid that is retained is buffered by
A. hemoglobin
B. plasma proteins
C. bicarbonate
D. bone
E. phosphate
REF. 7, p. 1566

165. The final correction of metabolic acidosis induced by acid infusion depends on
A. renal excretion of acid
B. respiratory excretion of carbonic acid
C. blood buffer
D. interstitial fluid buffers
E. cellular buffers
REF. 7, p. 1029

166. In acute respiratory alkalosis which of the following is true?
   A. Extracellular stores of sodium increase
   B. Extracellular stores of sodium decrease
   C. Extracellular stores of potassium increase
   D. Extracellular stores of chloride decrease
   E. Extracellular stores of lactate decrease
   REF. 7, p. 1576

167. The sole extracellular buffer mechanism in acute respiratory alkalosis is
   A. lactate
   B. carbonic acid
   C. chloride
   D. plasma proteins
   E. phosphate
   REF. 7, p. 1575

168. Posthypercapneic alkalosis is best treated by
   A. slowing respiratory rate
   B. potassium gluconate
   C. sodium chloride
   D. sodium bicarbonate
   E. observation
   REF. 7, p. 1576

169. Regarding posthypercapneic alkalosis, which of the following statements is correct?
   A. It is not accentuated by excessive use of diuretics
   B. It should be corrected by chloride administration
   C. The rate of the respirator should be increased
   D. Acetazolamide should be given
   E. Oxygen will correct the defect
   REF. 8, p. 148

170. Respiratory alkalosis is LEAST likely in which of the following?
   A. Psychogenic hyperventilation
   B. Salicylate intoxication
   C. Cirrhosis of the liver
   D. Cor pulmonale treated with diuretics
   E. Pneumonia
   REF. 8, p. 168

171. In which of the following situations is there a tendency for H^+ excretion to decrease?
A. Acute respiratory insufficiency
B. Diabetic ketoacidosis
C. Psychogenic hyperventilation
D. Pyloric stenosis and hypokalemia in an adult
E. Aldosterone excess
REF. 8, p. 166

172. Primary respiratory alkalosis may occur in all of the following EXCEPT
A. salicylate intoxication
B. assisted respiration
C. cirrhosis of the liver
D. acetazolamide administration
E. exercise
REF. 5, p. 207

173. Primary respiratory alkalosis is LEAST likely in which of the following?
A. Alveolar-capillary block syndromes
B. Anemia
C. Gram-negative bacteremia
D. Pneumothorax
E. Inspired carbon dioxide
REF. 5, p. 220

174. Which of the following features is LEAST likely to be present in severe metabolic alkalosis?
A. Tetany
B. Hyperventilation
C. Digitalis toxicity
D. Plasma volume contraction
E. Paralytic ileus
REF. 5, p. 216

175. Postoperative hypokalemic, hypochloremic alkalosis is usually the consequence of
A. dehydration secondary to tube feeding
B. acute renal failure
C. unrecognized diarrhea
D. nasogastric suction
E. hyperalimentation
REF. 5, p. 217

176. In a pure metabolic alkalosis if the serum HCO_3 is 34 mM, the PCO_2 should be
A. 20 mmHg
B. 30 mmHg
C. 40 mmHg
D. 60 mmHg
E. 70 mmHg
REF. 7, p. 1569

177. During gastric drainage all of the following occur EXCEPT
A. increased urine pH
B. decreased urine K
C. increased urine bicarbonate
D. decreased urine Cl
E. increased renin secretion
REF. 5, p. 1275

178. Metabolic alkalosis is LEAST likely in
A. severe diarrhea
B. pyloric stenosis
C. Bartter's syndrome
D. calcium carbonate administration
E. ethacrynic acid therapy
REF. 8, p. 145

179. In a pure metabolic acidosis, if the plasma HCO_3 is 14 mM, the PCO_2 should be
A. 52 mmHg
B. 40 mmHg
C. 28 mmHg
D. 10 mmHg
E. 18 mmHg
REF. 7, p. 1559

180. A patient has a PCO_2 of 70 mmHg and an arterial pH of 7.40. Which of the following statements is FALSE?
A. Diuretics have probably been given
B. The primary defect is a metabolic alkalosis
C. Cyanosis may be present
D. Cor pulmonale is a possible diagnosis
E. The plasma volume is probably contracted
REF. 8, p. 144

181. A cirrhotic patient has ascites, a hemoglobin level of 8 g/100 ml, PCO_2 of 40 mmHg, and pH of 7.55. Which of the following conditions is NOT likely to be present?
A. Folic acid deficiency
B. Mixed respiratory and metabolic alkalosis
C. Hypokalemia
D. Diuretic administration
E. Pure respiratory alkalosis
REF. 12(2), p. 162

182. A semicomatose patient with PCO_2 = 15 mmHg, Na = 140 mEq/L, HCO_3 = 13 mM, and Cl = 115 mEq/L is most likely to have
A. lactic acidosis
B. overcompensated respiratory alkalosis
C. severe diarrhea
D. diabetic ketoacidosis
E. aspirin overdosage
REF. 12(2), p. 34

183. A patient with chronic metabolic acidosis receiving alkali therapy may hyperventilate for several days after the acidosis is corrected. Which of the following findings would be most consistent with such a state?
A. pH 7.4, PCO_2 40, HCO_3 24
B. pH 7.5, PCO_2 40, HCO_3 30
C. pH 7.5, PCO_2 20, HCO_3 16
D. pH 7.3, PCO_2 30, HCO_3 14
E. pH 7.5, PCO_2 50, HCO_3 36
REF. 5, p. 226

184. A patient has a PCO_2 of 70 mmHg and a HCO_3 of 33 mM, which suggests
A. chronic respiratory acidosis
B. acute respiratory acidosis
C. respiratory and metabolic acute acidosis
D. respiratory acidosis and metabolic alkalosis
E. none of the above
REF. 7, p. 1557

185. The anion gap may be increased in
A. ammonium chloride intoxication
B. pyloric stenosis
C. bromide intoxication
D. multiple myeloma
E. cirrhosis of the liver
REF. 8, p. 122

186. A 45-year-old man with chronic cor pulmonale was admitted because of increasing dyspnea, cough, sputum, and "refractory" edema. PCO_2 is 60 mmHg and arterial pH 7.39. Which of the following statements is correct?
A. The patient has an uncomplicated respiratory acidosis
B. Potassium depletion is most unlikely
C. Immediate correction of the hypercapnia will restore acid-base balance
D. The patient has mixed respiratory acidosis and metabolic alkalosis
E. The patient should be treated with sodium bicarbonate
REF. 5, p. 226

187. In man, nitrogen is excreted in the urine in all of the following EXCEPT
A. uric acid
B. creatinine
C. urea
D. amino acids
E. ketone bodies
REF. 5, p. 43

188. Urea is formed from the cleavage of
A. ornithine
B. arginine
C. citrulline
D. succinic acid
E. fumaric acid
REF. 5, p. 47

189. Concerning the excretion of urea by the kidney, which of the following statements is FALSE?
A. A low-protein diet improves renal function and enhances the concentration ability of the kidney
B. The papillary portion of the collecting duct is moderately permeable to urea, and the permeability is increased by antidiuretic hormone
C. The cortical segment of the collecting duct is impermeable to urea
D. The distal convoluted tubule is impermeable to urea
E. The thin descending loop of Henle is moderately permeable to urea
REF. 6, pp. 424-425

190. Concerning the excretion of urea, which of the following statements is FALSE?
   A. A larger fraction of the filtered urea is reabsorbed during hydropenia
   B. Urea is reabsorbed from the medullary segment of the collecting duct
   C. The reabsorbed urea reenters the descending and thin ascending loops of Henle
   D. Urea transport is not affected by ADH
   E. Recirculation of urea is least during diuresis

   REF. 6, pp. 589-594

191. With respect to urea excretion, which of the following statements is FALSE?
   A. The urea clearance increases during diuresis up to flows of 3 ml/min
   B. The lower the urine to plasma ratio for creatinine, the lower the urea clearance
   C. At normal urine flows roughly 50% of the filtered urea is reabsorbed
   D. During antidiuresis more urea is reabsorbed from the collecting duct
   E. The percent of the filtered load of urea in the distal convoluted tubule exceeds that at the tip of the loop of Henle

   REF. 6, pp. 590-591

192. Which of the following statements about uric acid transport are FALSE?
   A. Uric acid is reabsorbed and secreted by the renal tubules
   B. Transport occurs mainly in the proximal portions of the nephron
   C. Changes in glomerular filtration are not a major determinant in regulating urate clearance
   D. With increasing urine flow, the urate clearance tends to rise
   E. Urate transport takes place mainly by diffusion

   REF. 6, pp. 621-623

193. In a large hospital population, the most common cause of hyperuricemia is likely to be
A. chronic renal insufficiency
B. inadequately treated hypertension
C. chronic treatment with diuretics
D. obesity and purine overingestion
E. adult-onset diabetes mellitus
REF. 7, p. 1222

194. Uric acid clearance is increased by which of the following?
A. Sulfinpyrazone
B. Angiotensin
C. Norepinephrine
D. Long-term thiazide diuretics
E. Respiratory acidosis
REF. 6, p. 625

195. Which of the following statements about uric acid transport are FALSE?
A. Uric acid concentration in the interstitium is highest in the juxtamedullary region
B. Uric acid transport in the proximal tubule is bidirectional
C. Hyperthyroidism increases the uric acid clearance
D. Pyrazinoate depresses mainly the secretion of uric acid
E. Acetazolamide in man slightly increases uric acid excretion
REF. 6, pp. 631-633

196. Serum uric acid levels tend to be lowest in association with which of the following?
A. Hypertriglyceridemia
B. Obesity
C. Treatment with high doses of aspirin
D. Chronic thiazide administration
E. Hyperparathyroidism
REF. 7, p. 1220

197. Impaired renal excretion is the cause of hyperuricemia in
A. psoriasis
B. lead poisoning
C. polycythemia vera
D. sickle cell disease
E. infectious mononucleosis
REF. 7, p. 831

198. Disproportionately high serum uric acid levels are LEAST likely in which of the following?
   A. Analgesic nephropathy
   B. Polycystic kidney disease
   C. Toxemia of pregnancy
   D. Hypertensive nephrosclerosis
   E. Lead nephropathy
   REF. 7, p. 1221

199. Clinical gout is LEAST likely to occur in
   A. sickle cell disease
   B. chronic lead poisoning
   C. Lesch-Nyhan syndrome
   D. chronic myeloid leukemia
   E. chronic renal failure
   REF. 7, p. 1222

200. Hypouricemia is most likely in which of the following?
   A. Generalized atherosclerosis
   B. Sarcoidosis
   C. Hypoparathyroidism
   D. Anaplastic lung cancer
   E. Aseptic necrosis of the femur
   REF. 6, p. 632

201. Which of the following statements about the Lesch-Nyhan syndrome is FALSE?
   A. Uric acid levels usually exceed 10 mg/100 ml
   B. Transmission is by a dominant gene
   C. Stones and renal failure are frequent
   D. Mental retardation, choreoathetosis and self-mutilation are characteristic
   E. Hypoxanthine-guanine phosphoribosyltransferase is absent
   REF. 7, p. 1219

202. Regarding the Lesch-Nyhan syndrome, which statement is FALSE?
   A. It affects boys
   B. The gene is carried on the X chromosome
   C. Tophi and gouty arthritis are common
   D. Patients usually present with athetosis
   E. Symptoms appear in the first weeks of life
   REF. 7, p. 1219

203. Hypouricemia occurs in
A. diabetes mellitus without glycosuria
B. diabetic ketoacidosis
C. diabetic nephropathy
D. Hodgkin's disease
E. none of the above
REF. 10, p. 1041

204. Large doses of salicylates in man with respect to urate causes
A. suppression of secretion only
B. suppression of reabsorption only
C. suppression of secretion and reabsorption
D. increased reabsorption and suppressed secretion
E. suppressed reabsorption and increased secretion
REF. 7, p. 1220

205. The hyperuricemia of chronic thiazide adminstration is most likely caused by
A. decreased glomerular filtration rate
B. decreased extracellular fluid volume
C. increased uric acid production
D. the underlying hypertension and the reduced renal plasma flow
E. increased lactate production
REF. 7, p. 1222

206. Which of the following is associated with a decreased urate clearance?
A. Inappropriate ADH secretion
B. Beta-hydroxybutyric acid
C. Estrogens
D. Probenecid
E. Mannitol
REF. 7, p. 1222

207. Hyperlactacidemia as a cause of hyperuricemia is LEAST likely in
A. fasting
B. toxemia of pregnancy
C. Down's syndrome
D. glycogen storage disease
E. diabetic ketoacidosis
REF. 7, p. 1221

208. Which of the following enzyme abnormalities does not cause hyperuricemia?
A. Phosphoribosylpyrophosphate amidotransferase
B. Hypoxanthine-guanine phosphoribosyltransferase
C. Phosphoribosylpyrophosphate synthetase
D. Glutathione reductase
E. Xanthine oxidase
REF. 7, p. 1218

209. Which of the following is true of glucose excretion by the kidney?
A. Depends only on glomerular filtration
B. Takes place by secretion in the proximal tubule
C. Is characterized by a sharp TmG at about 300 mg/min
D. Glucose does not appear in the urine until the filtered load is 50% greater than the reabsorptive capacity
E. Appearance of glucose in urine at low glucose blood levels depends on nephrons with high filtration rates to glucose reabsorptive capacity ratios
REF. 7, p. 1021

210. With regard to glucose reabsorption which statement is FALSE?
A. Glucose is reabsorbed by a limiting active transport rate
B. The carrier for glucose is unknown
C. Tubular transport maximum for glucose is roughly 300 mg/min
D. Phlorizin decreases the glucose/insulin ratio
E. Normally glucose is absent from the urine except for trace amounts
REF. 7, p. 1023

211. As dehydration is corrected in diabetic ketoacidosis, glycosuria will
A. increase
B. decrease
C. remain unchanged
D. decrease as blood glucose falls
E. disappear
REF. 5, p. 1342

212. Parathormone action on the tubule may result in
A. aminoaciduria
B. suppression of adenylcyclase
C. hypophosphaturia
D. hypomagnesuria
E. none of the above
REF. 5, p. 349

213. Which of the following physiologic effects suggests a proximal tubular site of action for a diuretic?
A. Significant phosphaturia
B. Depression of free water clearance
C. Hyperkalemia
D. A fractional bicarbonate excretion less than 0.2
E. Metabolic alkalosis
REF. 6, p. 1005

214. Which statement is FALSE regarding osmotic diuresis?
A. Urine flow and sodium excretion rise in proportion to to the osmotic load
B. During hydropenia the urine tends towards isotonicity
C. The initial event is probably interference with sodium reabsorption
D. Significant sodium loss occurs from the loop of Henle
E. The medullary concentration gradient is decreased
REF. 6, pp. 1008-1010

215. All but which of the following may play a role in the production of diuretic-induced hyponatremia?
A. Decreased glomerular filtration and increased proximal tubular sodium reabsorption
B. Decreased effective plasma volume and stimulation of antidiuretic hormone secretion
C. Hypoaldosteronism and increased migration of potassium into the cell
D. Decreased reabsorption of chloride and sodium in the distal convoluted tubule
E. Decreased delivery of filtrate to the distal diluting sites
REF. 8, p. 40

216. Which of the following statements apply to the effects of hypertonic saline or mannitol?
A. Free water reabsorption ($T^c H_2O$) tends to fall
B. Maximum attainable $T^c H_2O$ is 15 ml/min
C. Hydrochlorothiazide abolishes $T^c H_2O$
D. Measured $T^c H_2O$ invariably underestimates true water reabsorption from the collecting ducts
E. Decreased sodium transport in the ascending limb of the loop of Henle augments $T^c H_2O$
REF. 7, p. 1480

217. Regarding the antihypertensive effect of diuretics which of the following statements is FALSE?
A. Plasma renin levels are lowered
B. Cardiac output decreases
C. Extracellular fluid volume decreases
D. Peripheral resistance falls
E. Sensitivity to vasoconstrictor drugs decreases
REF. 10, p. 1114

218. Acetazolamide usually causes all but which of the following?
A. Alkaline urine
B. Bicarbonaturia
C. Kaliuresis
D. Decreased phosphate excretion
E. Decreased citrate excretion
REF. 6, p. 1011

219. Which of the following statements is FALSE regarding the effects of thiazide diuretics on potassium excretion?
A. The main effect is due to inhibition of potassium reabsorption in the proximal tubule
B. Potassium is added to the distal tubules by a diffusional process determined by the transtubular potential differences
C. Distal potassium secretion is enhanced by an increased rate of flow of fluid through the tubules
D. Potassium losses are difficult to replace by giving potassium supplements
E. Potassium supplements are most effective if not given simultaneously with the diuretic
REF. 7, p. 1601

220. All of the following reactions have been reported with thiazide diuretics EXCEPT
A. transient myopia
B. deafness
C. central disturbances of vision
D. agranulocytosis
E. thrombocytopenia
REF. 10, p. 1122

221. Which of the following statements is FALSE regarding the effect of thiazide diuretics on glucose metabolism?
A. Preexistent diabetes may be aggravated
B. Glucose tolerance may become impaired in nondiabetics
C. The level of circulating insulin is decreased and this may be due to potassium depletion
D. Peripheral utilization of glucose is increased
E. Treatment for hyperglycemia is rarely needed
REF. 10, p. 1175

222. Which of the following diuretics act on the proximal tubule?
A. Triamterene
B. Ethacrynic acid
C. Amiloride
D. Furosemide
E. Spironolactone
REF. 10, p. 1099

223. Impaired urinary dilution ability but preserved concentration ability suggests
A. thiazides
B. furosemide
C. mercurial diuretics
D. action on the medullary segment of the loop of Henle
E. action on proximal tubule
REF. 6, p. 1006

224. The main site of action of thiazide diuretics is the
A. thin segment of the loop of Henle
B. medullary pyramids
C. collecting duct
D. entire nephron
E. distal tubule
REF. 7, p. 1536

225. Which of the following diuretics inhibit active chloride reabsorption?
A. Amiloride
B. Mersalyl
C. Thiazides
D. Spironolactone
E. Triamterene
REF. 10, p. 1103

226. Metabolic alkalosis is a frequent complication of long-term diuretic therapy. Which of the following statements are true?
A. A urinary chloride concentration over 20 mEq/L suggests metabolic alkalosis secondary to diuretics
B. Bicarbonate loss and "secondary" plasma volume expansion perpetuate the maintenance of metabolic alkalosis
C. In most cases the administration of chloride cannot reestablish acid base equilibrium, because frequently potassium depletion perpetuates alkalosis
D. Coexistence of primary or secondary hyperaldosteronism would prevent the development of metabolic alkalosis
E. Massive doses of spironolactone will only partially prevent diuretic-induced alkalosis and hypokalemia
REF. 7, p. 1570

227. Regarding the effects of diuretics on urate metabolism, which of the following statements is FALSE?
A. The hyperuricemia is probably due to contraction of the extracellular space
B. Repletion of the extracellular volume raises uric acid excretion to its normal level
C. Intravenously administered chlorothiazide has a uricosuric action
D. The hyperuricemia can be overcome with allopurinol or probenecid
E. The reduced extracellular volume acts to promote increased urate reabsorption in the distal tubule
REF. 14(2), pp. 203, 246

228. Regarding diuretic-induced metabolic alkalosis, which of the following statements is true?
   A. Compensation is achieved by partial stimulation of the respiratory center
   B. An increase of 1 mEq/L in plasma bicarbonate raises arterial PCO_2 by 0.9 mmHg
   C. Metabolic alkalosis is best tolerated by patients with respiratory insufficiency
   D. Effective treatment involves chloride restriction and the provision of adequate potassium
   E. Chloride restriction lowers PCO_2 and improves cyanosis and the other symptoms

   REF. 7, p. 1567

229. Regarding the treatment of diabetes insipidus, which of the following statements is FALSE?
   A. Thiazides may have a direct vasopressin-like effect on renal tubules
   B. The main effect of thiazides is to produce chronic extracellular volume contraction, with diminished delivery of sodium to the diluting sites
   C. Thiazides decrease free water clearance by acting on the cortical segment of the ascending loop of Henle
   D. Thiazides are ineffective in nephrogenic diabetes insipidus because their action requires presence of small amounts of ADH
   E. Thiazide therapy is contraindicated in diabetes insipidus

   REF. 10, p. 1118

230. Which of the following does NOT produce antidiuresis in high doses in diabetes insipidus?
   A. Hydrochlorothiazide
   B. Chlorthalidone
   C. Furosemide
   D. Ethacrynic acid
   E. Spironolactone

   REF. 10, p. 1118

231. Which of the following diuretics increases K^+ excretion in the urine?
   A. Amiloride
   B. Triamterene
   C. Mercurials
   D. Spironolactone
   E. Acetazolamide

   REF. 10, p. 428

232. Which of the following drugs is NOT contraindicated in advanced renal failure?
A. Furosemide
B. Spironolactone
C. Triamterene
D. Amiloride
E. Wax-embedded potassium tablets
REF. 10, p. 1121

233. Theophylline acts as a diuretic by all of the following mechanisms EXCEPT
A. increasing renal blood flow
B. increasing GFR
C. increasing free water clearance
D. increasing Na excretion
E. decreasing filtration fraction
REF. 10, p. 306

234. Which of the following diuretics would NOT increase natriuresis following a maximum dose of ethacrynic acid?
A. Furosemide
B. Hydrochlorothiazide
C. Mercurial compound
D. Acetazolamide
E. None of the above
REF. 7, p. 796

235. Chronic thiazide administration may cause all of the following EXCEPT
A. hypomagnesuria
B. hypocalciuria
C. hypouricuria
D. hypokalemia
E. alkalosis
REF. 10, p. 602

236. Ethacrynic acid has all of the following properties EXCEPT
A. it decreases free water clearance
B. carbonic anhydrase inhibition
C. it decreases free water resorption
D. it causes hypokalemia
E. it results in systemic alkalosis
REF. 5, p. 673

237. A maximal fractional sodium excretion of 20% or over has been observed with which of the following diuretics?
 A. Acetazolamide
 B. Hydrochlorothiazide
 C. Meralluride (Mercuhydrin)
 D. Chlorthalidone
 E. Spironolactone
 REF. 6, p. 1004

238. Mercurial diuretics increase the excretion of all of the following EXCEPT
 A. chloride
 B. bicarbonate
 C. calcium
 D. magnesium
 E. potassium
 REF. 5, p. 670

239. Which of the following is the major mechanism by which mercurials act as diuretics?
 A. Increase of free water clearance
 B. Decrease in reabsorption of chloride in the collecting duct
 C. Decrease in chloride reabsorption in the ascending limb
 D. Decrease in Na reabsorption in the distal tubule
 E. Combination with protein-bound sulfydryl groups in the loop of Henle
 REF. 5, p. 671

240. Which of the following statements about furosemide is FALSE?
 A. Furosemide at maximal doses is more effective than thiazide diuretics
 B. The drug is effective even at very low filtration rates
 C. Renal blood flow and glomerular filtration are increased, unless there is considerable hypovolemia
 D. The ability of the kidneys to elaborate a concentrated urine is maintained
 E. Other diuretics may potentiate its effect
 REF. 2, p. 796

241. In the treatment of pulmonary edema with intravenous furosemide, which of the following statements is true?
   A. The effect of furosemide depends largely on its systemic blood pressure-reducing action
   B. A direct relation has been shown between relief of symptoms and the onset of diuresis
   C. A reduction in left ventricular and end-diastolic pressure may be the main effect
   D. The main effect is by potentiating the renal effect of intravenous aminophylline
   E. Tourniquets are contraindicated when IV furosemide is given
   REF. 10, p. 1110

242. Prolonged usage of furosemide can result in all of the following EXCEPT
   A. hypokalemia
   B. hypochloremia
   C. hypomagnesemia
   D. hypocalcemia
   E. bicarbonaturia
   REF 5, p. 673

243. Furosemide inhibits
   A. chloride transport in the ascending limb
   B. potassium transport in the distal tubule
   C. sodium transport in the collecting duct
   D. chloride transport in the proximal tubule
   E. chloride transport in the collecting duct
   REF. 5, p. 671

244. Which of the following effects is less frequently observed with ethacrynic acid than with furosemide?
   A. Gout
   B. Gastrointestinal hemorrhage
   C. Deafness
   D. Diabetes
   E. Hypokalemia
   REF. 10, p. 1124

245. Furosemide
   A. inhibits carbonic anhydrase enzyme profoundly
   B. inhibits ATPase activity of renal tubule
   C. enhances diuretic activity by acidosis
   D. decreases excretion of titratable acidity
   E. inhibits diuretic activity by hypochloremia
   REF. 10, p. 1103

246. Characteristics of triamterene include which of the following?
   A. Decreased glomerular filtration
   B. Inhibition of aldosterone action on tubule
   C. Rapid induction of diuresis
   D. Action at the loop of Henle
   E. Decreased bicarbonate excretion
   REF. 10, p. 1106

247. Full natriuretic action of spironolactone is evident
   A. within 10 to 30 min
   B. within 2 to 4 hours
   C. 12 to 20 hours
   D. in a few days
   E. none of the above
   REF. 10, p. 1110

248. With regard to the effect of spironolactone, which of the following statements is FALSE?
   A. The excretion of potassium is depressed
   B. The excretion of bicarbonate is enhanced
   C. Uric acid retention is unusual
   D. Urinary concentrating ability is abolished
   E. Gynecomastia and impotence may occur
   REF. 10, p. 1126

2. CLINICAL EVALUATION OF RENAL FUNCTION

DIRECTIONS: Each of the questions or incomplete statements below is followed by five suggested answers or completions. Select the one that is best in each case.

---

249. A 35-year-old man has long-standing nonpitting edema of the extremities. He has lived most of his life in the tropics. He gives a history of passing milky urine. The cause of the abnormal appearance of the urine is
  A. lipiduria
  B. urinary tract infection
  C. gonorrhea
  D. chyluria
  E. drinking excessive amounts of milk
  REF. 1, p. 440

250. A 25-year-old woman was admitted to the hospital in an unconscious state. There were no relatives, friends, or witnesses to provide a history. The bladder was catheterized and a centrifuged urine specimen contained fat droplets that rose to the top. The patient is most likely suffering from
  A. eclampsia
  B. fractures
  C. carbon monoxide poisoning
  D. all of the above
  E. none of the above
  REF. 1, p. 440

251. Autoregulation of renal blood flow maintains a constant GFR despite changes in perfusion pressure. Autoregulation does not depend on renal nerves, vasopressor substances, or renal sympathetic tone under basal conditions. Thus a patient overtaken by fright or pain will have
A. no change in renal blood flow (RBF)
B. no change in GFR
C. fall in RBF
D. fall in GFR
E. fall in RBF and GFR
REF. 1, p. 445

252. A 15-year-old boy was found to have the nephrotic syndrome. Renal biopsy disclosed minimal-change disease. Creatinine clearance determined from a timed specimen of urine while the patient remained supine was found to be 150 ml/L. The cause of the elevated creatinine clearance is
A. increased permability of glomerular capillary surface
B. inadequate urine collection
C. decreased glomerular plasma oncotic pressure
D. increased renal blood flow
E. increased transcapillary hydrostatic pressure
REF. 1, p. 445

253. Isosmolar urine is usually found in
A. acute tubular necrosis
B. hepatorenal syndrome
C. acute glomerulonephritis
D. volume depletion
E. after infusion urography
REF. 2, p. 1600

254. Normally many factors determine the passage of proteins through the glomerular capillary wall. In glomerular disease albuminuria is a frequent finding. What is the cause of the increased loss of albumin in the urine?
A. Increase in glomerular epithelial pore size
B. Change in molecular configuration of albumin
C. Change in electric charge of albumin
D. Change in deformability of albumin
E. Loss of glomerular polyanion
REF. 1, p. 446

255. Disproportionate impairment of the concentrating ability of urine occurs in
A. hypercalcemic nephropathy
B. acute glomerulonephritis
C. chronic glomerulonephritis
D. a normal person consuming a high-protein diet
E. embolism of the renal artery
REF. 2, p. 1659

256. An increase of the urinary specific gravity out of proportion to the expected osmolality would NOT occur in which of the following?
A. Severe proteinuria
B. Contrast media from pyelography
C. Detergents used to clear the hydrometer
D. Testing urine at body temperature
E. Glycosuria
REF. 7, p. 60

257. A 26-year-old woman is admitted to the hospital for investigation of the nephrotic syndrome. The relative clearances of proteins of increasing molecular weights were determined and this disclosed a dominance of albumin and absence of higher molecular weight globulins. Which of the following conditions does this finding favor?
A. Membranous glomerulopathy
B. Proliferative glomerulonephritis
C. Minimal-change disease
D. Membranoproliferative glomerulonephritis
E. Focal glomerulonephritis
REF. 1, p. 461

258. The occurrence of a vasopressin (Pitressin)-resistant hyposthenuria is LEAST likely in which of the following?
A. Obstructive uropathy
B. Focal nephritis
C. Sarcoidosis
D. Amyloid
E. Hypokalemic nephropathy
REF. 7, p. 58

259. Defects in concentrating ability with preservation of diluting capacity are seen in all of the following EXCEPT
A. sickle cell disease
B. hypokalemia
C. adrenal insufficiency
D. hyperparathyroidism
E. medullary cystic disease
REF. 7, p. 1498

260. Which of the following values for normal 24-hour solute excretions are INCORRECT?
A. Uric acid: 600 mg
B. Urea nitrogen: 11 g
C. Creatinine: 6 g
D. Hydrogen ions: 60 mEq
E. Potassium: 50 to 100 mEq
REF. 7, p. 46

261. A patient has a serum Na^+ of 135 mEq/L; serum Cl^- of 104 mEq/L; serum glucose of 180 mg%, BUN of 28 mg%; uric acid of 8 mg%. The calculated serum osmolality is
A. 360
B. 239
C. 290
D. 312
E. 300
REF. 10, p. 94

262. In the presence of a blood urea nitrogen (BUN) of 70 mg%, which of the following statements regarding a concentration test is FALSE?
A. The test is of little clinical value
B. The dehydration may involve some risk to the patient
C. The patient cannot concentrate because the remaining nephrons are in a state of osmotic diuresis
D. The specific gravity will be at least 1.003
E. A normal urinary concentration ability may be expected after the administration of vasopressin
REF. 7, p. 62

263. A 35-year-old man was found to have proteinuria on routine physical examination. Electrophoresis of urinary protein disclosed a large amount of low-molecular-weight proteins and relatively slight increase in the excretion of albumin. Radioimmunoassay disclosed a predominance of $beta_2$-microglobulins. The cause of the proteinuria is

A. cadmium poisoning
B. mercury intoxication
C. penicillamine toxicity
D. glomerulonephritis
E. none of the above

REF. 1, p. 461

264. Normally creatinine clearance provides a good clinical measure of glomerular filtration rate despite the fact that some creatinine is secreted by the proximal tubule, because creatinine is overestimated by calorimeter as a result of measuring some noncreatinine chromogen as well. In patients with moderate renal failure, however, creatinine clearance overestimates glomerular filtration rate. The overestimate is because

A. creatinine secretion increases and noncreatinine chromogen rises less
B. creatinine secretion increases and noncreatinine chromogen remains high as in normal renal function
C. creatinine secretion decreases and noncreatinine chromogen decreases
D. creatinine secretion decreases and noncreatinine chromogen remains high as in normal renal function
E. none of the above

REF. 1, p. 462

265. In clinical practice the most frequent error in the measurement of creatinine clearance is

A. not correcting for creatinine secretion
B. not collecting adequate urine
C. not correcting for noncreatinine chromogen
D. not accounting for variation in endogenous creatinine production
E. none of the above

REF. 1, p. 463

266. Although blood urea nitrogen is frequently used as a measure of glomerular filtration rate it is both imperfect and less reliable than plasma creatinine concentration. All of the following contribute to its unreliability EXCEPT
A. urea production is variable and is dependent on hepatic function and dietary conditions
B. urea reabsorption varies with the state of hydration
C. in renal failure urea secretion by the tubules predominates
D. in renal failure blood urea nitrogen concentration is influenced by protein in the diet
E. bleeding in the gut increases blood urea nitrogen
REF. 1, p. 463

267. A 47-year-old man with diabetes mellitus became oliguric after an intravenous pyelogram. Urine osmolality was found to be 480 mOsm. The most likely diagnosis in this patient is
A. acute renal failure
B. prerenal azotemia
C. papillary necrosis
D. diabetic nephropathy
E. obstructive uropathy
REF. 1, p. 463

268. Inulin is used to measure the glomerular filtration rate because it is
A. handled in the same way as creatinine
B. completely removed during one passage through the kidney
C. filtered but not reabsorbed or secreted
D. filtered and secreted but not reabsorbed
E. filtered and reabsorbed but not secreted
REF. 7, p. 46

269. Which of the following is usually NOT associated with large or normal size kidneys in renal disease?
A. Diabetes
B. Amyloid
C. Scleroderma
D. Acute tubular necrosis
E. Chronic pyelonephritis
REF. 10, p. 1611

270. Maximal urine-concentrating ability is measured by restricting fluid intake. All of the following end points will provide maximal urine concentrating ability EXCEPT
A. the patient loses at least 3% body weight
B. three consecutive urine specimens show no further increase in osmolality
C. 16 hours of fluid restriction
D. less than 16 hours fluid restriction in patients with severe inability to conserve water
E. the patient loses at least 1% body weight
REF. 1, p. 463

271. The maximum diluting capacity of the kidney is assessed by the rapid administration of 1200 ml of water by mouth to a fasting subject. The measurement that will best achieve the maximum diluting capacity is
A. osmolality less than 80 mOsm in at least one of three hourly urine specimens
B. urine volume should exceed 900 ml at 3 hours
C. the peak rate of urine flow should be at the second hour
D. all of the above
E. none of the above
REF. 1, p. 463

272. Both maximal diluting and maximal concentrating ability of the kidney may be impaired by all of the following EXCEPT
A. furosemide
B. ethacrynic acid
C. glycosuria
D. fasting
E. mannitol
REF. 1, p. 463

273. The urine of healthy individuals is generally more acid than body fluids because of the endogenous production and renal excretion of nonvolatile acids. Which of the following forms of acid excretion is neglibible?
A. Ammonium
B. Free hydrogen ion
C. Titratable acid
D. All of the above
E. None of the above
REF. 1, p. 463

274. In patients with chronic renal failure and small contracted kidneys, renal biopsy examination is
A. mandatory after preliminary dialysis
B. absolutely contraindicated
C. usually quite helpful
D. occasionally permissible but relatively hazardous
E. mandatory if transplantation is being contemplated
REF. 7, (2nd ed.), p. 204

275. A patient with severe hypertension and normal serum creatinine level is found to have 4 g proteinuria/24 hr. On pyelography the right kidney is large (16 cm) and the left one small (7 cm) and poorly outlined. Arteriography shows possible right renal artery stenosis. The most appropriate next investigation would be
A. bilateral retrograde pyelography
B. right percutaneous renal biopsy
C. left percutaneous renal biopsy
D. right "open" surgical renal biopsy
E. bilateral renal vein renin determinations
REF. 7, pp. 1374-1375

276. A 30-year-old woman presents with severe hypertension of acute onset, bilateral papilledema, considerably impaired renal function (BUN 150 mg%), and 1 g proteinuria/24 hr. She says that she is allergic to contrast media and refuses permission for retrograde pyelography or ultrasonography. Which of the following statements is the most appropriate?
A. Open renal biopsy should be done after the blood pressure is controlled
B. Renal biopsy may be safely attempted provided the bleeding time is normal
C. Biopsy is not necessary because bilateral nephrectomy will be required anyhow
D. Renal biopsy is unsafe in any event
E. Renal biopsy may be performed provided the patient is first adequately dialyzed
REF. 7 (2nd ed.), p. 204

277. A low complement level is seen in all but which of the following?
A. Membranous glomerulonephritis
B. Mesangiocapillary glomerulonephritis
C. Bacterial endocarditis
D. Shunt nephritis
E. Systemic lupus erythematosus
REF. 7, p. 554

278. White cell casts in acute poststreptococcal glomerulonephritis are most likely to be
A. evidence of streptococcal infection
B. superimposed pyelonephritis
C. contamination from the lower urinary tract
D. consistent with acute exudative glomerulonephritis
E. the result of aspirin overdosage
REF. 7, p. 75

279. An elderly patient is admitted to the hospital from the nursing home in a stuporous state with volume contraction and hypotension. Urinary sodium is less than 10 mEq/L. This finding is diagnostic of
A. Addison's disease
B. hyperaldosteronism
C. sodium-losing nephritis
D. extrarenal sodium loss
E. inappropriate secretion of ADH
REF. 1, p. 464

280. A decreasing rate of protein excretion in a patient with stable renal function indicates which of the following?
A. Amyloidosis is almost certainly present
B. A pattern rarely seen in membranous glomerulopathy
C. The serum albumin may have decreased
D. The glomerular damage may be worsening
E. Urinary obstruction is a serious consideration
REF. 7, p. 71

281. A 32-year-old black man with a blood pressure of 200/160 mmHg has a strong family history of hypertension. At the age of 12 he had an episode of facial swelling and bloody urine. His 24-hour urinary protein excretion is 450 mg and the BUN level is 10 mg/100 ml. Which of the following statements is the most appropriate?
A. The patient is certain to have essential hypertension
B. Latent glomerulonephritis is highly unlikely
C. Renal biopsy should be performed without delay
D. Treatment with antihypertensive drugs should be started without delay, and the urine reexamined later
E. Retrograde pyelography will clinch the diagnosis
REF. 7, pp. 76, 734

282. A 24-year-old jogger was admitted to the hospital with a history of acute oliguria. The urine sodium was 40 mEq/L. This finding is consistent with all of the following EXCEPT
A. acute renal failure
B. incomplete urinary obstruction
C. prerenal azotemia
D. furosemide
E. ethacrynic acid
REF. 1, p. 464

283. A 25-year-old woman was admitted to the hospital for evaluation of metabolic alkalosis. The urine chloride concentration was greater than 10 mEq/L. This finding is consistent with all of the following EXCEPT
A. vomiting
B. diuretics
C. severe K depletion
D. Bartter's syndrome
E. Cushing's syndrome
REF. 1, p. 464

284. The tetrabromophenol blue-impregnated paper test (dip-stick) gives a false-positive reaction for protein in which of the following conditions?
A. Urine collected after urography
B. High-dose penicillin therapy
C. When urine is very turbid
D. All of the above
E. None of the above
REF. 13, p. 306

285. A 72-year-old woman develops oliguria following resection of an aortic aneurism which had involved both renal arteries. A fluid load and furosemide are given and urine output increases to 100 ml/hour. Which of the following statements applies best?
A. The patient had "transient" acute tubular necrosis
B. The urinary sodium concentration before furosemide was given was 60 mEq/L
C. The urine to plasma urea concentration was 20:1
D. The administration of furosemide was ill-advised
E. Anticoagulants were responsible for the development of this syndrome
REF. 7, p. 188

286. A 49-year-old man was admitted for evaluation of proteinuria. An intravenous pyelogram was planned as part of the evaluation. Which of the following conditions is LEAST likely to precipitate reduction in renal function after IVP?

A. Diabetes mellitus
B. Hypouricemia
C. Multiple myeloma
D. Volume contraction
E. Preexisting azotemia

REF. 1, p. 465

3. HYPERTENSION

DIRECTIONS: Each of the questions or incomplete statements below is followed by five suggested answers or completions. Select the one that is best in each case.

---

287. A 45-year-old black man with no other known risk factors has a blood pressure of 140/95 (phase 4). At the end of 6 months observation, the most appropriate approach is to
   A. start treatment using propranolol
   B. start treatment with potassium chloride
   C. start diuretic treatment and restrict sodium intake
   D. determine phase 5 diastolic blood pressure
   E. use a large cuff and order an EKG
   REF. 9, p. 17

* 288. Concerning blood pressure measurement which of the following is true?
   A. The arm should be at the level of the heart and if not supported the diastolic pressure may decrease by as much as 10%
   B. If a difference is noted in the arms, the lower arm is probably the most accurate
   C. Standing diastolic pressure is usually lower than supine in patients with mild hypertension
   D. The initial reading is usually lower than subsequent readings
   E. A pressure difference between the two arms may signify a subclavian steel syndrome
   REF. 9, p. 19

¥ 289. The most likely cause for erratic blood pressure control is
A. failure to prescribe a diuretic
B. poor drug absorption
C. noncompliance
D. faulty sphygmomanometer
E. all of the above
REF. 9, p. 175

290. Which of the following statements concerning hypertension is FALSE?
A. When diastolic blood pressure is above 90 mmHg life expectancy is significantly reduced at all ages and in both sexes
B. The official criteria for the World Health Organization define normotension as systolic blood pressure 140-160 mmHg and diastolic blood pressure 90 mmHg to 95 mmHg
C. The rate of rise in blood pressure is higher in individuals with a higher starting blood pressure
D. Women tolerate hypertension better than do men
E. Hypertension affects 15-20% of all adult Americans
REF. 9, pp. 2-5

291. In patients with borderline hypertension which of the following statements is true?
A. Cardiac output is usually increased
B. Blood volume is usually increased
C. Peripheral vascular resistance is markedly elevated
D. The alpha adrenergic nervous system is dominant
E. These patients usually have a poor response to beta blockers
REF. 9, p. 12

292. Most epidemiological studies conclude the following EXCEPT
A. renovascular disease occurs in 0.05% of hypertensives
B. pheochromocytoma occurs in 0.2% of hypertensives
C. essential hypertension occurs in 89-95% of hypertensives
D. chronic renal disease is the etiology for 2-5% of hypertension
E. none of the above
REF. 9, p. 14

293. Which of the following blood pressure ranges are defined as "borderline hypertension" in the young adult?
A. 140/90 to 160/95
B. 120/80 to 140/90
C. 120/80 to 165/90
D. 130/85 to 140/95
E. 130/85 to 139/89
REF. 9, p. 2

294. Blood pressure may increase with
A. obesity
B. high alcohol intake
C. cigarette smoking
D. gout
E. all of the above
REF. 9, pp. 26-29

295. Which of the following statements is FALSE concerning hypertensive blacks as compared to hypertensive whites?
A. Blacks tend to have lower plasma renins
B. Blacks tend to have lower renal kallikrein excretion
C. Blacks have a better response to beta blockers
D. Blacks tend to have a greater response to diuretics
E. Blacks tend to have lower dopamine hydroxylase activity
REF. 9, p. 73

296. Stress
A. may raise blood pressure by activation of the sympathetic nervous system
B. is high in air traffic controllers who have a high economic status and low incidence of hypertension
C. may raise blood pressure by stimulating cortisol production
D. may lead to hyperperfusion nephropathy by increasing renal blood flow
E. is higher among high socioeconomic groups
REF. 9, p. 65

DIRECTIONS: For each of the questions or incomplete statements below, one or more of the answers or competions given is correct. Select

(A) if only 1, 2, and 3 are correct
(B) if only 1 and 3 are correct
(C) if only 2 and 4 are correct
(D) if only 4 is correct
(E) if all are correct

---

297. With a sphygmomanometer, a blood pressure of 190/90 is obtained in an otherwise well 82-year-old man. Which of the following statements is/are true?
   1. One should begin therapy cautiously with small doses of antihypertensives
   2. Once-a-day dosage with guanethidine 50 mg qod, should be considered for convenience and compliance in a forgetful elderly patient
   3. Actual blood pressure may be lower
   4. Actual blood pressure may be higher

   REF. 9, p. 14

298. Less than 1% of the hypertensive population have
   1. Cushing's disease
   2. primary aldosteronism
   3. pheochromocytoma
   4. renovascular hypertension

   REF. 2, p. 1477

299. A 25-year-old woman who is not taking any medication known to cause hypertension has, for the fourth visit, a blood pressure of 170/120. Physical examination reveals no abnormalities but
   1. she should be reassured that women suffer less from the complications of hypertension than men
   2. the patient should be started on a high-potassium diet and seen again in 6 months
   3. red blood cell sodium should be measured
   4. the patient should be investigated for secondary hypertension

   REF. 2, p. 1481

Directions Summarized

(A) 1, 2, 3 only; (B) 1, 3 only; (C) 2, 4 only; (D) 4 only; (E) all

---

300. A thin patient with a sinus bradycardia is consistently found to have a blood pressure of 170/100 mmHg by one observer and 160/100 mmHg by another observer. Cause of this discrepancy includes
    1. using too wide a cuff
    2. digit preference of individual observers changing silent gap
    3. changing silent gap
    4. different rates of deflation by the two observers

    REF. 9, p. 20

301. On fundoscopy which abnormalities are seen in both hypertension and arteriosclerosis?
    1. Increased light reflex
    2. Narrowed caliber of vessels
    3. A-V crossing defects
    4. Copper wiring

    REF. 9, p. 34

302. Which of the following statements is true concerning the prevalence of hypertension?
    1. About 60 million Americans have chronic elevation of blood pressure
    2. Five million Americans have borderline hypertension
    3. Patients with blood pressure of 90 to 104 mmHg have an increased risk of premature death
    4. Because of an increasing awareness by the public and medical professionals that the prevalence of heart attack, stroke, and renal failure is increased, a large proportion of patients have their blood pressure lowered properly in the United States

    REF. 9, pp. 1-11

* 303. A 50-year-old man comes to your office. For the second time his blood pressure is 160/100. After a careful history and physical examination, which tests would be appropriate to obtain?
1. Plasma catecholamine levels, chest x-ray
2. Blood chemistries including serum creatinine, potassium, uric acid, and glucose levels
3. Plasma renin activity and serum calcium
4. Urinalysis and electrocardiogram

REF. 9, p. 30

DIRECTIONS: Each of the questions or incomplete statements below is followed by a list of suggested answers or completions. Select the one that is best in each case.

---

304. According to Guyton's hypothesis on regulation of blood pressure, which of the following is LEAST important in immediate pressure control?
A. Peripheral resistance of arterioles
B. Cardiac output
C. Venous compliance
D. Baroreceptors
E. Renal fluid volume mechanism

REF. 12(8), p. 15

305. Natriuretic response to sodium load is observed in all of the following EXCEPT
A. hypertensive subjects
B. normotensive subjects whose blood pressure is elevated with metaraminol
C. normotensive subjects with pulmonary hypertension
D. acute water load in hypertensive subjects
E. hypertensive subjects with lowering of elevated blood pressure

REF. 9, p. 51

306. Concerning most patients with essential hypertension, which of the following statements is FALSE?
    A. Plasma volume at one time was probably initially expanded
    B. Plasma volume when measured is usually lower than in normal subjects
    C. Plasma volume is usually inappropriately elevated for the degree of blood pressure elevation
    D. Plasma volume is usually lower in obese hypertensives than in nonobese hypertensives
    E. Interstitial volume is probably expanded
    REF. 9, pp. 47-48

307. With resetting of the pressure natriuresis curve in essential hypertension all of the following occur EXCEPT
    A. filtration fraction decreases with decreased renal blood flow
    B. glomerular filtration is usually well maintained but renal plasma flow is decreased
    C. filtration fraction increases and glomerular filtration is normal
    D. filtration fraction is increased and renal blood flow is decreased
    E. filtration fraction decreases and glomerular filtration is normal
    REF. 9, p. 49

308. In red cells of patients with essential hypertension, the following transport defects have been described EXCEPT
    A. intracellular Na content is increased
    B. K-Na countertransport is increased with an increased K efflux
    C. passive Na influx is increased
    D. Na-K cotransport is increased with increased efflux of Na
    E. increased rate of Na-Li cotransport
    REF. 9, p. 57

309. Concerning natriuretic hormone, which of the following is true?
   A. It is thought to be responsible for the exaggerated natriuresis in hypertensives when given an acute sodium load
   B. Its effect is thought to be inhibition of the Na, K-dependent ATPase which is responsible for the influx of sodium in extrusion of potassium from cells
   C. The source of this hormone is thought to be the adrenals
   D. It causes the highest rate of natriuresis in volume contracted patients with high plasma renin activity
   E. It is found in highest levels in Addisonian rats
   REF. 9, p. 56

310. In essential hypertension
   A. serum sodium is high
   B. serum sodium is low
   C. urinary sodium is high
   D. urinary sodium is low
   E. sodium in the vessel wall is high
   REF. 9, p. 57

311. In essential hypertension blood flow is increased to the
   A. muscle
   B. kidney
   C. liver
   D. gut
   E. brain
   REF. 1, p. 140

312. In essential hypertension intracellular
   A. calcium is probably elevated
   B. magnesium is probably elevated
   C. potassium is probably elevated
   D. calcium is probably low
   E. sodium is probably low
   REF. 9, p. 61

313. Concerning the carotid sinus and aortic arch baroreceptor activity which of the following statements is FALSE?
   A. Complete denervation in animals causes persistent hypertension
   B. In essential hypertension baroreceptor sensitivity may be slightly reduced
   C. Baroreceptor activity may be increased in young borderline hypertensives
   D. With decreased baroreceptor activity, one may see an exaggerated rise in peripheral resistance and diastolic blood pressure during upright tilting
   E. Higher pressures are needed to activated baroreceptors in hypertensives

   REF. 9, p. 67

314. The hyperuricemia of early essential hypertension is most likely due to which of the following?
   A. Hyperlactacidemia
   B. Reduced GFR
   C. Reduced renal blood flow
   D. Hyperreninemia
   E. Decreased filtration fraction

   REF. 9, p. 27

315. Hormones that directly control blood pressure in man include all of the following EXCEPT
   A. epinephrine
   B. norepinephrine
   C. renin
   D. vasopressin
   E. aldosterone

   REF. 10, pp. 650-661

316. Catecholamines produce all of the following effects EXCEPT
   A. apprehension followed by hyperventilation, palpitations, and tremor
   B. sustained rise of systolic pressure
   C. increased cardiac output
   D. increased muscle blood flow
   E. increased renal blood flow

   REF. 12(8), p. 109

317. Which of the following statements is FALSE regarding PGI_2?
A. Causes peripheral arteriolar vasodilation
B. Is metabolized by the lung
C. Is a potent natriuretic
D. Stimulates renin release
E. Has a negative chronotropic effect
REF. 12(8), p. 183

318. Kallikrein excretion is decreased in patients with
A. essential hypertension
B. pheochromocytoma
C. primary aldosteronism
D. all of the above
E. none of the above
REF. 12(8), p. 179

319. Angiotensin infusion to a normotensive subject results in all of the following EXCEPT
A. elevation of glomerular filtration rate
B. reduction of renal salt excretion
C. reduction of renal blood flow
D. antidiuresis
E. increase in prostaglandin production
REF. 10, pp. 657-658

320. Regarding angiotensin I, which of the following statements is true?
A. It is the most powerful vasoconstrictor known to man
B. It is acted upon in the liver by converting enzymes
C. It is made up of ten amino acids
D. It stimulates aldosterone release
E. It is formed from "big renin"
REF. 10, pp. 657-658

321. Which of the following statements about angiotensin II is FALSE?
A. It is a peptide composed of eight amino acids
B. It acts as a constrictor of the arterioles
C. Under certain conditions it causes sodium retention
D. Under certain conditions it causes natriuresis
E. During volume contraction it acts on the adrenal to suppress aldosterone secretion
REF. 10, p. 677

322. Which of the following statements about angiotensinogen (renin substrate) is FALSE?
    A. It is made mainly in the liver
    B. Its concentration is sharply increased after bilateral adrenalectomy
    C. Its concentration does not fall after bilateral nephrectomy
    D. Its concentration is decreased in cirrhosis of the liver
    E. Its concentration is increased by estrogen
    REF. 10, pp. 652-653

323. Which of the following maneuvers does NOT stimulate release of renin?
    A. Application of venous tourniquets
    B. Quiet standing
    C. Intravenous furosemide
    D. Indomethacin
    E. Metolazone
    REF. 10, p. 671

324. Which of the following mechanisms would suppress renin release?
    A. Decreased pressure within the renal afferent arteriole
    B. High concentration of sodium or chloride within the macula densa
    C. Stimulation of the renal sympathetic nerves
    D. Hyperkalemia
    E. Epinephrine
    REF. 9, pp. 214-217

325. Which of the following is NOT an action of angiotensin II?
    A. Contraction of vascular smooth muscle
    B. Stimulation of aldosterone secretion
    C. Suppression of thirst
    D. Increase in secretion of catecholamines
    E. Stimulation of the vasomotor center
    REF. 9, p. 222

326. Increased plasma renin activity is expected in which of the following conditions?
    A. Congenital adrenal hyperplasia
    B. Autonomic dysfunction
    C. Androgen therapy
    D. Cushing's syndrome
    E. Estrogen therapy
    REF. 9, p. 228

327. Administration of saralasin results in an initial increase of blood pressure followed by a rapid decline in a hypertensive patient both before and after salt depletion. Most likely this hypertension is
A. neurogenic in origin
B. volume dependent
C. associated with high plasma renin
D. labile
E. factitious
REF. 9, pp. 280-281

328. Abnormally high angiotensinogen (renin substrate) levels are found in which of the following conditions?
A. A patient on estrogen therapy
B. Hodgkin's disease
C. Colitis
D. Essential hypertension
E. Leukemia
REF. 9, p. 213

329. Aldosterone is always increased in
A. essential hypertension
B. malignant hypertension
C. pheochromocytoma
D. Liddle's syndrome
E. polycystic kidney
REF. 9, p. 293

X 330. In which of the following conditions is the secretion of aldosterone reduced?
A. Malignant hypertension
B. Addison's disease
C. Nephrotic syndrome
D. Bilateral adrenal hyperplasia
E. Liver cirrhosis
REF. 9, p. 862

331. The main abnormality in the arteriolonephrosclerosis seen with aging is
A. fibrinoid necrosis
B. intimal hyalinization
C. medial hypertrophy
D. intimal proliferation
E. medial cystic degeneration
REF. 10, p. 1693

332. Renin levels are most commonly determined by
A. measurement of angiotensin I generation
B. radioimmune assay of renin
C. radioimmune assay for renin substrate
D. rate of aldosterone secretion
E. angiotensin II levels
REF. 9, p. 226

333. Which lesion is LEAST consistent with "benign" nephrosclerosis?
A. Hyalinization of the afferent arterioles
B. Interstitial fibrosis
C. Shrinkage and hypocellularity of the glomerular tuft
D. Proliferation of fibroblasts derived from connective tissue
E. Appearance of an homogeneous material internal to Bowman's capsule
REF. 10, pp. 1691-1694

334. Histologic changes of nephrosclerosis include all of the following EXCEPT
A. wrinkled thickened glomerular capillary walls
B. periglomerular fibrosis
C. loss of foot processes
D. tubular atrophy
E. altered elastic lamella
REF. 10, p. 1693

335. The thrombosis that forms atheroma is initiated primarily by
A. platelets
B. fibrin
C. lipid
D. fibroblasts
E. cholesterol
REF. 2, p. 1468

336. Arteriosclerosis
A. occurs only in hypertension
B. is the cause of hypertension
C. does not affect the efferent glomerular arterioles
D. most extensively involves the kidneys
E. affects only the efferent glomerular arteriole
REF. 2, pp. 1662-1663

DIRECTIONS: Each set of lettered headings below is followed by a list of numbered words or phrases. For each numbered word or phrase select

(A) if the item is associated with A <u>only</u>
(B) if the item is associated with B <u>only</u>
(C) if the item is associated with <u>both</u> A and B
(D) if the item is associated with <u>neither</u> A nor B

A. Constant blood flow but varying vascular resistance
B. Resistance changes match blood flow and metabolic needs
C. Both
D. Neither

337. Skeletal muscle
338. Kidneys
339. Brain
REF. 12(8), p. 15

Match the following effect with the substance

A. Hypertensive
B. Hypotensive
C. Both
D. Neither

340. Vasopressin
341. Prostaglandins
342. Renin
343. Aldosterone
344. Glucagon
345. Bradykinin
REF. 12(8), p. 224

DIRECTIONS: Each of the questions or incomplete statements below is followed by five suggested answers or completions. Select the one that is best in each case.

---

346. Which of the following types of hypertension is NOT due to mineralocorticoid excess?
    A. Adrenocortical carcinoma
    B. 11 beta hydroxylase deficiency
    C. Liddle's syndrome
    D. 17 alpha hydroxylase deficiency
    E. 11 Desoxycorticosterone administration
    REF. 9, p. 306

347. Suppressed plasma renin is always found in which of the following?
    A. Essential hypertension
    B. Coarctation of the aorta
    C. Pheochromocytoma
    D. Conn's syndrome
    E. Cushing's syndrome
    REF. 10, p. 280

348. Hypertension in renal allotransplantation may be due to all of the following EXCEPT
    A. renal artery stenosis
    B. chronic rejection
    C. corticosteroid therapy
    D. renin production by the native kidney
    E. azothioprine therapy
    REF. 9, p. 291

349. Which of the following patients is likely to develop a change in mental status?
    A. A previously normotensive 40-year-old man admitted with a headache and blood pressure of 180/130
    B. A known hypertensive who rarely takes medication with blood pressure 180/132
    C. A new hypertensive admitted with blood pressure of 190/140 is started on diazoxide; blood pressure is lowered to 110/70
    D. A patient with a cerebral infarction, admitted with hypertension; blood pressure is lowered to 105/70 with nitroprusside
    E. All of the above
    REF. 9, p. 197

350. The most common cause of cerebral hemorrhage in hypertension is
A. atheroma
B. berry aneurysms
C. Charcot-Bouchard aneurysms
D. rupture of the arteriosclerotic vessels
E. hemorrhage following thrombosis
REF. 2, p. 1479

351. Renal biopsy in a patient with severe hypertension, papilledema, mild proteinuria, and renal failure is LEAST likely to show
A. glomerular proliferation
B. focal necrotizing glomerulonephritis
C. margination of leukocytes
D. arteriolar hyaline
E. fibrinoid material and polymorphonuclear cells in the walls of the arterioles
REF. 10, pp. 1696-1699

352. In primary malignant nephrosclerosis all but which of the following are found?
A. Proliferative endarteritis of the afferent arterioles
B. Proliferative endarteritis of the small interlobular arteries
C. Diffuse proliferative glomerulonephritis
D. Necrotizing arteriolitis
E. Necrotizing glomerulitis
REF. 10, pp. 1696-1699.

353. A patient with sudden onset of monocular blindness, acute pancreatitis, and renal failure is likely to have
A. polyarteritis nodosa
B. obstructive uropathy
C. acute tubular necrosis
D. artheroembolic renal disease
E. acute glomerulonephritis
REF. 10, p. 1747

354. A 32-year-old man with paroxysmal hypertension and headaches but repeatedly normal VMA, catecholamine, and metanephrine determinations in the urine and plasma should be evaluated for
A. cerebral astrocytoma
B. nonfunctioning adrenal tumor
C. coarctation of the aorta
D. aberrant adrenal tissue
E. incomplete urine collections
REF. 9, p. 341

355. Which of the following may distinguish between hypertension from idiopathic causes and eclampsia?
A. Serum creatinine
B. Proteinuria
C. Serum uric acid
D. Urinary sediment
E. GFR
REF. 9, p. 374

356. A woman in her twenty-fourth week of pregnancy has a blood pressure of 170/100 mmHg. This blood pressure should be considered
A. borderline to mild
B. pseudohypertension of pregnancy
C. hyperkinetic syndrome
D. severe
E. low
REF. 12(8), p. 203

357. When treating a patient with pheochromocytoma which of the following drugs or combinations are best avoided?
A. Dibenzaline
B. Beta blocker prior to alpha blocker
C. Alpha blocker prior to beta blocker
D. Prazosin
E. Clonidine
REF. 9, p. 355

358. Which one of the following tests is likely to be abnormal in a patient with neurofibromatosis and hypertension?
A. 24-hour urine for metanephrine
B. Plasma renin activity
C. Serum cortisol
D. 24-hour urine for aldosterone
E. Fractional excretion of potassium
REF. 9, p. 344

359. Orthostatic hypotension, diabetes, hypermetabolism, and hyperparathyroidism are suggestive of
A. Cushing's syndrome
B. essential hypertension
C. malignant hypertension
D. pheochromocytoma
E. cerebellar hemangioblastoma
REF. 9, p. 346

360. Which of the following substances FALSELY elevate the urine vanillylmandelic acid (VMA) level?
A. Methyldopa
B. Monoamine oxidase inhibitors
C. Clofibrate
D. Ethanol
E. Nitroglycerine
REF. 9, p. 350

DIRECTIONS: For each of the questions or incomplete statements below, one or more of the answers or completions given is correct. Select
(A) if only 1, 2, and 3 are correct
(B) if only 1 and 3 are correct
(C) if only 2 and 4 are correct
(D) if only 4 is correct
(E) if all are correct

---

361. Which of the following characterizes hypertension in a patient with endstage renal disease?
1. Usually volume related
2. Plasma renin is usually low
3. Can usually be controlled with adequate ultrafiltration
4. Is associated with a low plasma volume
REF. 9, p. 242

362. A 14-year-old boy who had a sore throat 2 weeks ago presents with a blood pressure of 140/100. Which might be the most appropriate test?
1. Urinary sediment examination
2. Urine culture
3. Urine examination with sulfosalicylic acid
4. Urine pH
REF. 1, p. 1632

363. A 10-year-old boy has a blood pressure of 160/60 mmHg. Which diagnosis should be considered?
1. Hyperthyroidism
2. Anemia
3. Aortic coarctation
4. Arteriovenous fistula
REF. 9, p. 13

Directions Summarized

(A) 1, 2, 3 only; (B) 1, 3 only; (C) 2, 4 only; (D) 4 only; (E) all

---

364. A 30-year-old woman with severe hypertension has a systolic and diastolic midabdominal bruit. Which of the following screening tests might be appropriate?
   1. Depressor response to saralasin infusion
   2. Upright plasma renin activity
   3. Adrenal angiography
   4. Intravenous urography

   REF. 2, p. 1481

365. Which of the following statements applies to the hypertensive state in which one renal artery is clipped and the other kidney is removed?
   1. Plasma renin levels tend to be low
   2. The hypertension is largely volume dependent
   3. Total body sodium is high
   4. The plasma volume is contracted

   REF. 9, pp. 261-262

366. Which of the following are associated with systolic hypertension?
   1. Aortic insufficiency
   2. Thyrotoxicosis
   3. Beriberi
   4. Rigidity of the aorta

   REF. 9, p. 13

367. In a patient who is hypokalemic from diuretics, which of the following results would make primary aldosteronism likely?
   1. Urine sodium 120 mEq/24-hr and urine potassium 12 mEq/24 hr
   2. Urine sodium 200 mEq/24-hr and urine potassium 20 mEq/24 hr
   3. Urine sodium 120 mEq/24-hr and urine potassium 20 mEq/24 hr
   4. Urine sodium 80 mEq/24-hr and urine potassium 40 mEq/24 hr

   REF. 9, p. 200

368. Which of the following tests would be most helpful in localizing an aldosterone-producing adenoma that is 15 mm in size?
1. Adrenal photoscanning
2. Adrenal venography
3. Retroperitoneal CT scan
4. Adrenal vein aldosterone levels

REF. 9, pp. 308-310

369. In a 34-year-old presenting with hypertension, frontal headaches, polydipsia, and paresthesias, which of the following tests would be most helpful?
1. Palpation of the femoral arteries
2. Plasma renin
3. Echocardiogram
4. Plasma potassium

REF. 9, p. 298

370. Fibrinoid necrosis is
1. usually present in essential hypertension
2. present only in the media
3. affects only the intima
4. usually present in malignant hypertension

REF. 9, p. 197

371. A renal biopsy in a patient with severe hypertension, papilledema, mild proteinuria, and renal failure may show
1. glomerular proliferation
2. focal necrotizing glomerulonephritis
3. arteriolar hyaline
4. margination of leukocytes

REF. 10, pp. 1696-1699

372. A 32-year-old man with paroxysmal hypertension and headaches, but repeatedly normal VMA, catecholamine, and metanephrine determinations in the urine and plasma should be evaluated for
1. incomplete urine collections
2. aberrant adrenal tissue
3. nonfunctioning adrenal tumor
4. cerebral astrocytoma

REF. 9, p. 341

Directions Summarized

(A) 1, 2, 3 only; (B) 1, 3 only; (C) 2, 4 only; (D) 4 only; (E) all

---

373. Renal and nonrenal causes of accelerated hypertension may be differentiated by
   1. presence of proteinuria
   2. presence of RBC casts
   3. high serum creatinine
   4. none of the above

   REF. 10, pp. 1479, 1637

374. Arthromatous stenosis of the renal artery
   1. usually involves the proximal one-third of the renal artery
   2. may be bilateral
   3. often shows poststenotic dilatation
   4. may appear as a string of beads

   REF. 10, pp. 1724-1725

375. A volume-dependent hypertension associated with excess sodium and water may occur in which of the following?
   1. Primary aldosteronism
   2. Licorice-induced hypertension
   3. Chronic renal failure with fluid retention
   4. After bilateral nephrectomy

   REF. 9, p. 228

376. Which of the following is/are true of fibromuscular dysplasia?
   1. May be unilateral or bilateral
   2. May occur at extrarenal sites
   3. The distal two-thirds of arteries characteristically may be involved
   4. May be associated with intracranial aneurysm

   REF. 10, pp. 1725-1727

377. Which of the following statement(s) is/are true?
   1. Red wine may interfere with the action of MAO inhibitors
   2. Naloxone may cause hypotension in patients taking nontricyclic antidepressants
   3. Nonsteroidal antiinflammatory drugs may interfere with the action of diuretics and beta blockers
   4. Nose drops may cause hypotension

   REF. 9, p. 406

378. A patient presents with palpitation, headache, and signs of sodium retention. Which antihypertensive(s) may he have been taking?
1. Hydralazine
2. Phentolamine
3. Minoxidil
4. Sotalol
REF. 9, pp. 161-163

379. Beta receptors are blocked by
1. ergot alkaloids
2. nicotine
3. phentolamine
4. propranolol
REF. 9, p. 147

380. Which of the following statement(s) concerning prazosin is/are true?
1. It may be useful in pheochromocytoma
2. It is contraindicated in pheochromocytoma
3. It is a postsynaptic alpha-adrenergic receptor blocker
4. One should start with high doses in the morning
REF. 9, pp. 145-146

381. Which antihypertensive(s) act(s) to increase plasma renin activity?
1. Methyldopa
2. Guanabenz
3. Clonidine
4. Captopril
REF. 9, pp. 166-167

382. A 60-year-old diabetic woman with a blood pressure of 160/105 mmHg carries the diagnosis of hyporeninemic hypoaldosteronism. Which of the following diuretics would be best avoided to treat her hypertension?
1. Metolazone
2. Amiloride
3. Chlorthalidone
4. Aldactone
REF. 9, p. 132

Directions Summarized

(A) 1, 2, 3 only; (B) 1, 3 only; (C) 2, 4 only; (D) 4 only; (E) all

383. A 60-year-old woman who has been taking digoxin is given a diuretic when seen in an emergency room for shortness of breath. One month later she returns complaining of syncope. Which might be appropriate in this patient?
1. Obtain an EKG
2. Start nifedipine
3. Check serum potassium
4. Check serum calcium and magnesium

REF. 9, p. 1217

384. Which of the following statement(s) is/are true concerning calcium channel blockers?
1. Verapamil and nifedipine block the entry of calcium into the cells
2. Diltiazem increases calcium's exit from the cells
3. Heart failure has been reported in patients given calcium channel blockers who are also receiving beta blockers
4. Sublingual nifedipine has an immediate effect lasting about 3 hours

REF. 9, p. 166

385. Somnolence is an outstanding side effect of
1. methyldopa
2. hydralazine
3. clonidine
4. guanethidine

REF. 9, p. 139

386. Failure of ejaculation occurs with
1. reserpine
2. methyldopa
3. nifedipine
4. guanethidine

REF. 9, p. 137

387. Nitroprusside has which of the following actions?
1. Dilates systemic veins
2. Reduces venous return
3. Reduces afterload by reducing peripheral resistance
4. Increases cardiac output in patients not in heart failure

REF. 9, p. 203

388. Which of the following statement(s) concerning antihypertensives is/are true?
1. Chlorthalidone, metolazone, and trimterene are all diuretics and have similar effects on potassium balance
2. Captopril, tepratide, and saralasin are angiotensin-converting enzyme inhibitors
3. Lipid soluble beta blockers include propranolol, timolol, and atenolol
4. Minoxidil, hydralazine, diazoxide, and nitroprusside are vasodilators and may all increase plasma renin activity

REF. 9, p. 121

389. A patient with a blood pressure of 160/110 mmHg has been started on guanethidine 12. 5 mg daily. The following day his blood pressure is 160/105. What should be done?
1. Increase the dose of guanethidine to 50 mg daily and see the patient in 1 month
2. Obtain a plasma renin
3. Restrict sodium intake and increase potassium intake
4. Continue observation for another week if the patient is not symptomatic

REF. 9, pp. 135-137

390. According to the step care program
1. one may start with a thiazide diuretic or a beta blocker
2. clonidine might be an appropriate second-step drug
3. prazosin may be used as a second- or third-step drug
4. minoxidil should be reserved for patients with refractory hypertension

REF. 2, pp. 1485-1486

391. Which agent(s) may increase renal blood flow?
1. Propranolol
2. Atenolol
3. Timolol
4. Nadolol

REF. 9, p. 156

Directions Summarized

(A) 1, 2, 3 only; (B) 1, 3 only; (C) 2, 4 only; (D) 4 only; (E) all

392. Which statement(s) is/are true concerning beta blockers?
   1. May cause hyperkalemia
   2. Have been associated with hyporeninemia
   3. May interfere with insulin release
   4. Are contraindicated in the presence of hypokalemia

   REF. 9, pp. 157-160

DIRECTIONS: Each group of questions below consists of five lettered headings followed by a list of numbered words or statements. For each numbered word or statement, select the one lettered heading that is most closely associated with it. Each lettered heading may be selected once, more than once, or not at all.

For each antihypertensive match the physiologic action

A. Increased venous capacitance
B. Sympathetic blockade
C. Converting enzyme inhibition
D. Volume depletion
E. Alpha blockade with short duration of action

393. Nitroprusside
394. Captopril
395. Methyldopa
396. Amiloride
397. Phentolamine
398. Chlorthalidone

REF. 9, p. 121

For each region indicate the expected outcome

A. Lesions in the nucleus of the solitary tract (NTS)
B. Lesions in the area surrounding the anteroventral third ventricle (AV3V)
C. Lesions of the restiform body
D. Lesion of the nucleus of V
E. Lesions of the nucleus cuneatus

399. Lead to hypertension in animals
400. Prevent the development of hypertension in animals
401. Possible origin of natriuretic hormone
REF. 9, pp. 67, 68

Match the appropriate drug with the paradoxical response

A. Guanethidine
B. Propranolol
C. Pindolol
D. Saralasin
E. Clonidine

402. Withdrawal, followed by increased catecholamine (rebound)
403. Stimulation of angiotensin receptors
404. Intrinsic sympathomimetic activity
405. Unopposed alpha adrenergic vasoconstriction
406. Releases catecholamines when given intravenously
REF. 9, p. 406

Match the appropriate diagnosis with the urinary protein and intravenous urographic findings

A. Nephrosclerosis
B. Chronic glomerulonephritis
C. Chronic pyelonephritis
D. Renovascular disease
E. Conn's syndrome

407. 24-hour protein, 3.8 g, normal intravenous urogram
408. 24-hour protein 400 mg, normal intravenous urogram
409. 24-hour protein 400 mg, intravenous urogram shows distorted calyces with symmetrical contraction
410. 24-hour protein 800 mg, intravenous urogram shows a 7 cm L kidney and a 10 cm R kidney
REF. 9, p. 244

DIRECTIONS: Each set of lettered headings below is followed by a list of numbered words or phrases. For each numbered word or phrase select

(A) if the item is associated with A only
(B) if the item is associated with B only
(C) if the item is associated with both A and B
(D) if the item is associated with neither A nor B

Match the appropriate diagnosis with the urinary protein and intravenous urographic findings.

A. 11 hydroxylase deficiency
B. 3-B-dehydrogenase deficiency
C. Both
D. Neither

411. Hypertension
412. Hypokalemia
413. Hyperkalemia
414. Treated with glucocorticoids
415. Treated with metapyrone
416. Hypogonadism
417. Virilization
418. Usually fatal in childhood
REF. 9, pp. 400-406

A. Bilateral nodular hyperplasia
B. Adrenal aldosterone-producing adenoma
C. Both
D. Neither

419. Associated with hypokalemia, hypertension, and suppression of plasma renin
420. More common in men than in women
421. Plasma aldosterone levels fall in upright posture
422. Plasma aldosterone levels do not fall in upright posture
423. Adrenal venous sampling shows bilateral abnormality
424. Associated with hypotension
REF. 9, p. 292

4. DEVELOPMENTAL, VASCULAR, TUBULAR, AND NEOPLASTIC LESIONS

DIRECTIONS: Each of the questions or incomplete statements below is followed by five suggested answers or completions. Select the one that is best in each case.

---

425. Which of the following is NOT characteristic of the nail patella syndrome?
A. Proliferative glomerulonephritis
B. Iliac horns
C. Fibrils in the glomerular basement membrane
D. Autosomal dominant inheritance
E. Subluxation of radial heads
REF. 10, p. 1546

426. Familial juvenile nephronophthisis is identical with
A. medullary sponge kidney
B. medullary cystic disease
C. chronic interstitial nephritis
D. chronic pyelonephritis
E. polycystic disease of the kidneys
REF. 7, p. 1147

427. Patients with medullary cystic disease have
A. generally an asymptomatic course
B. cysts mainly in the cortex
C. progressive renal failure
D. enlarged kidneys
E. diagnosis made by intravenous pyelography
REF. 7, p. 1149

428. Which of the following features is rare in medullary sponge kidney?
A. Recurrent hematuria
B. Recurrent nephrolithiasis
C. Recurrent urinary tract infection
D. Anemia
E. Abnormal IVP
REF. 1, p. 592

429. Foam cells may be found in all of the following conditions EXCEPT
   A. chronic glomerulonephritis
   B. lipoid nephrosis
   C. membranous glomerulonephritis
   D. hereditary nephritis
   E. nephrosclerosis
   REF. 7, p. 1169

430. Which of the following most strongly suggests unilateral agenesis of the kidney?
   A. Enlargement of the contralateral kidney
   B. Absent kidney shadow on one side of IVP
   C. Urinary concentration defect
   D. GFR below 60 ml/min
   E. Hemitrigone on cytoscopy
   REF. 1, p. 593

431. Which of the following is NOT seen with nephroptosis?
   A. Ureteral colic in an upright posture
   B. Postural hypertension
   C. Postural hyperaldosteronism
   D. Ureteral colic relieved by the Trendelenburg position
   E. Renal failure
   REF. 1, p. 593

432. All of the following may be presenting features of renal vein thrombosis EXCEPT
   A. severe lumbar pain
   B. ureteral notching on intravenous pyelography
   C. hematuria
   D. proteinuria
   E. medial deviation of the ureter
   REF. 2, p. 1664

433. Renal vein thrombosis may be a complication of all of the following EXCEPT
   A. hypernephroma
   B. congestive heart failure
   C. terminal patient with papillary necrosis
   D. nephrosclerosis
   E. nephrotic syndrome
   REF. 2, p. 1664

434. In paroxysmal nocturnal hemoglobinuria
   A. red cells are destroyed in the reticuloendothelial system
   B. hemolysis occurs at night even if the patient sleeps during the day
   C. blood transfusions aggravate the hemolysis
   D. hemolysis is unrelated to plasma pH
   E. death occurs from arterial thrombosis
   REF. 1, p. 1870

435. The initial renal damage in disseminated intravascular coagulation is
A. hyaline thrombi
B. swelling of endothelial cells
C. crescent formation
D. disruption of the basement membrane
E. mesangial cell proliferation
REF. 7, p. 294

436. Which of the following is a long-term complication of the hemolytic-uremic syndrome of infancy?
A. Anemia
B. Thrombocytopenia
C. Hypertension
D. Intravascular coagulation
E. None of the above
REF. 3, p. 910

437. The renal biopsy appearance of glomerular capillary and arteriolar "hyaline" thrombi is LEAST compatible with
A. acute anuric renal failure
B. thrombocytopenic purpura
C. arthralgia and pleuritic pain
D. dysuria and sulfonamide therapy
E. microangiopathic hemolytic anemia
REF. 13, p. 444

438. Microangiopathic hemolytic anemia is LEAST likely in
A. systemic lupus erythematosus
B. thrombotic thrombocytopenic purpura
C. hemolytic-uremic syndrome
D. Henoch-Schönlein purpura
E. malignant hypertension
REF. 7, p. 1283

439. Occlusion of renal arterioles by needle-shaped clefts, with fibrous organization and marginal recanalization, is most consistent with
A. headache, arthritis, and sudden blindness in an elderly patient who has a raised sedimentation rate
B. dysphagia, Raynaud's phenomenon, hypertension, and acute renal failure
C. sudden monocular blindness, gastrointestinal bleeding, and renal failure in a 70-year-old man
D. arthralgia, pleurisy, and hypergammaglobulinemia in a young woman with a positive serological test for syphilis
E. arthralgia, eosinophilia, sudden footdrop, and hypertension
REF. 7, p. 1391

440. Sex-linked dominant mode of inheritance occurs in
A. Wilson's disease
B. cystinuria
C. cystinosis
D. Hartnup disease
E. vitamin D-resistant rickets
REF. 7, p. 1055

441. Which of the following is transmitted as an autosomal dominant character?
A. Lowe's syndrome
B. Wilson's disease
C. Primary renal tubular acidosis (RTA)
D. Nephrogenic diabetes insipidus
E. Fanconi's syndrome
REF. 7, p. 1040

442. Which of the following diseases is NOT transmitted as an autosomal character?
A. Vitamin D-resistant rickets
B. Cystinosis
C. Cystinuria
D. Galactosemia
E. Primary hyperoxaluria
REF. 7, p. 1055

443. A specific defect of transport systems both in the renal tubules and the jejunum has been described in all of the following EXCEPT
A. cystinuria
B. hypercalciuria
C. Hartnup disease
D. Wilson's disease
E. some cases of prolinuria
REF. 7, p. 991

444. In Fanconi's syndrome urinary proteins consist mainly of
A. globulins
B. albumin
C. albumin and globulins
D. alpha-2-globulins
E. macroglobulins
REF. 7, p. 68

445. Which of the following substances are found in urine of patients with Hartnup disease?
A. Glucose
B. Phosphate
C. Protein
D. Tryptophan
E. Cystine
REF. 3, p. 1573

446. In Hartnup disease which of the following amino acids are NOT found in the urine?
A. Histidine
B. Tryptophan
C. Phenylalanine
D. Asparagine
E. Arginine
REF. 7, p. 993

447. In proximal renal tubular acidosis which of the following is NOT true?
A. There is a reduced maximal, proximal reabsorption of bicarbonate
B. The distal acidification system is intact
C. With ammonium chloride administration urine pH falls below 5.4
D. There is excess bicarbonate in the urine
E. The distal acidifcation is impaired
REF. 7, p. 1039

448. Patients with proximal renal tubular acidosis will have an acid urine if
A. serum bicarbonate is low
B. serum chloride is low
C. serum potassium is low
D. serum sodium is low
E. none of the above
REF. 5, p. 898

449. Which of the following conditions causes proximal rather than distal tubular acidosis?
A. Hyperglobulinemia
B. Lowe's disease
C. Analgesic nephropathy
D. Fructose intolerance
E. None of the above
REF. 7, p. 1073

450. Match the following
1. Hartnup disease
2. Lowe's syndrome
3. Vitamin D-resistant rickets
4. Distal renal tubular acidosis
5. Renal glycosuria

A. Phosphaturia only
B. Cataracts
C. No clinical abnormality
D. Pellagra rash
E. Renal calculi
REF. 3, p. 1572

451. Ceramide trihexosidase deficiency is found in
A. hereditary nephritis
B. familial hyperprolinemia
C. Fabry's disease
D. Fanconi's syndrome
E. oxaluria
REF. 7, p. 1178

452. Mental retardation, renal ectasia, seizures, and renal fibrosis occur in
A. Fabry's disease
B. familial hyperprolinemia with renal disease
C. hereditary nephritis
D. Hartnup disease
E. Lignac Fanconi's syndrome
REF. 7, p. 1007

453. Hepatoma commonly occurs in
A. Wilson's disease
B. tyrosinemia
C. cystinosis
D. cystinuria
E. Hartnup disease
REF. 7, p. 1072

454. A pellagrous skin lesion is found in
A. cystinuria
B. cystinosis
C. Hartnup disease
D. Wilson's disease
E. oxaluria
REF. 7, p. 1003

455. Which of the following is true for nephrogenic diabetes insipidus?
A. It is inherited as autosomal dominant inheritance
B. It is inherited as autosomal recessive character
C. The GFR is low
D. Serum ADH is low
E. Female heterozygotes frequently exhibit a diminished concentration ability
REF. 7, p. 1073

456. Nephrogenic diabetes insipidus is unlikely to be encountered in
A. obstructive uropathy
B. chronic pyelonephritis
C. medullary cystic disease
D. nephrocalcinosis
E. acute glomerulonephritis
REF. 2, p. 610

457. Hypernephroma arises from the
A. glomerular epithelial cell
B. tubular epithelial cell
C. epithelial cells of the pelvicalyceal system
D. glomerular endothelial cell
E. juxtaglomerular apparatus
REF. 1, p. 595

458. A 40-year-old man was found to have a solitary coin lesion in the lung, elevated serum alkaline phosphatase and $alpha_2$ globulin, high ESR, and was subsequently found to have a hypernephroma of the kidney. Which of the following treatments is justified?
A. No treatment as the patient has evidence of metastases in the lungs and liver
B. Nephrectomy
C. Irradiation to kidney and lungs
D. Irradiation and actinomycin D therapy
E. None of the above
REF. 1, p. 595

5. PROTEINURIA, GLOMERULONEPHRITIS, AND THE NEPHROTIC SYNDROME

DIRECTIONS: Each of the questions or incomplete statements below is followed by a list of suggested answers or completions. Select the one that is best in each case.

---

459. Which of the following gives a false positive test for protein with the sulphosalicylic acid test?
    A. Aspirin
    B. Tetracycline
    C. Tolbutamide
    D. Alphamethyl dopa
    E. Indomethacin
    REF. 7, p. 65

460. Microscopical hematuria is LEAST common in
    A. minimal change disease (lipoid nephrosis)
    B. membranous glomerulonephritis
    C. proliferative glomerulonephritis
    D. membranoproliferative glomerulonephritis
    E. lupus nephritis
    REF. 13, p. 338

461. Regarding the urinary sediment, which of the following statements is FALSE?
    A. White cells disintegrate in alkaline urine
    B. Red cell casts indicate glomerular injury
    C. Trauma or exercise can produce red cell casts
    D. Maltese crosses are seen in acute glomerulonephritis
    E. The presence of red cells should always be viewed with suspicion
    REF. 13, pp. 305, 308, 311

462. Concerning protein excretion in normal subjects, which of the following statements is FALSE?
    A. Daily excretion is usually less than 150 mg
    B. Urinary protein concentration rarely exceeds 10-20 mg/100 ml
    C. At least 80% of the normal urinary protein is albumin
    D. About 25 mg Tamm-Horsfall protein are excreted daily
    E. The Dipstix is insensitive to light chain protein
    REF. 7, pp. 62-65

463. Which of the following statements is true about paper strip urinalysis methods?
    A. More accurate than precipitation tests
    B. More specific for globulins
    C. False positive reactions do not occur
    D. False negative reactions are frequent
    E. Cannot be used to detect Bence Jones proteins
    REF. 7, p. 64

464. Which of the following statements regarding Tamm-Horsfall protein is FALSE?
    A. It is a mucoprotein
    B. It is a component of hyaline casts
    C. It is secreted in the distal nephron
    D. Its detection indicates tubular disease
    E. It is precipitated in acid urine
    REF. 7, p. 64

465. The nephrotic syndrome could be seen in all of the following EXCEPT
    A. right-sided heart failure
    B. constrictive pericarditis
    C. obstruction of the inferior vena cava above the renal veins
    D. polycystic renal disease
    E. amyloidosis
    REF. 7, pp. 771-772

466. Regarding renal vein thrombosis (RVT), which of the following statements is correct?
A. Unilateral RVT with ipsilateral proteinuria has not been observed clinically
B. RVT may cause a sudden deterioration of renal function in adults
C. Anticoagulation always leads to recanalization of the renal vein and improvement in renal function
D. Experimental increase of venous pressure in animals causes a nephrotic syndrome
E. None of the above is correct
REF. 7, pp. 771-772

467. RVT could be seen in association with which of the following conditions?
A. SLE
B. Amyloidosis
C. MGN
D. MPGN
E. All of the above
REF. 7, pp. 771-772

468. Which of the following is the single most important criterion for the diagnosis of the nephrotic syndrome?
A. Edema
B. Serum albumin under 3 g/dl
C. Urinary protein more than 3. 5 g/24 hr
D. Hypercholesterolemia
E. Hypercoagulability
REF. 10, p. 1407

469. Regarding the nephrotic syndrome, which of the following statements is correct?
A. Increased proximal tubular reabsorption of protein
B. Increased proximal tubular catabolism of protein
C. Increased hepatic synthesis of protein
D. All of the above
E. None of the above
REF. 7, p. 773

470. In the hyperlipidemia of the nephrotic syndrome, which of the following statements is correct?
   A. There is no correlation between hypoalbuminemia and hypercholesterolemia
   B. HDL increase with severe hypoalbuminemia
   C. Increased VLDL causes lactescense of nephrotic serum
   D. LDL increase with severe nephrotic syndrome
   E. Accelerated atherosclerosis is definitely established
   REF. 7, pp. 784, 790-791

471. In the nephrotic syndrome which of the following statements is FALSE?
   A. Fanconi's syndrome may be caused by tubular damage
   B. Serum 25-OH-Vit D is increased
   C. Serum T_4 is decreased
   D. Serum ionized Ca^{++} is decreased
   E. Patients are clinically euthyroid
   REF. 7, p. 788

472. In the nephrotic syndrome which of the following statements is correct?
   A. IgG is increased
   B. IgA is increased
   C. IgM is increased
   D. T-lymphocyte dysfunction is invariable
   E. All of the above statements are correct
   REF. 7, p. 789

473. Regarding the GBM, which of the following statements is FALSE?
   A. Molecules greater than 40,000 daltons are normally filtered
   B. The slit pores between the epithelial cells probably prevent filtration of large molecules
   C. The polyanion glycoprotein may repel albumin
   D. All of the above are false
   E. None of the above is false
   REF. 7, pp. 774-775

474. Regarding the nephrotic syndrome, which of the following statements is FALSE?
   A. Albumin synthesis is probably 120% of normal
   B. Absolute rate of albumin catabolism is increased
   C. Edema is due to a decrease in plasma oncotic pressure
   D. Plasma volume by current measurements is normal or increased in most patients
   E. Some studies have shown decreased Na absorption by the proximal convoluted tubule

   REF. 7, pp. 777-783

475. Regarding coagulation defects in nephrotic syndrome, which of the following statements is FALSE?
   A. Most consistent abnormality is an increase in fibrinogen
   B. Plasminogen is almost always decreased
   C. Factor V is increased
   D. Platelet aggregation is enhanced
   E. Plasma fibrinogen level and turnover are related to degree of hypoalbuminemia

   REF. 7, p. 789

476. Regarding orthostatic proteinuria, which of the following statements is FALSE?
   A. There is normal protein excretion on recumbency
   B. A minority of patients subsequently have persistent proteinuria
   C. Most patients eventually lose considerable renal function
   D. 24-hour urine protein is rarely more than 1 g
   E. None of the above is false

   REF. 7, p. 70

477. Which of the following is NOT a cause of nephrotic syndrome?
   A. Trimethadione
   B. Quinidine
   C. Gold salt
   D. EDTA
   E. Intravenous drug abuse

   REF. 10, p. 1437

478. Which of the following is LEAST likely to cause a nephrotic syndrome?
A. Glomerulonephritis
B. Polycystic renal disease
C. Renal vein thrombosis
D. Lupus nephritis
E. Kimmelsteil-Wilson syndrome
REF. 7, p. 769

479. Nephritogenic immune complexes form in which of the following conditions?
A. Antibody excess
B. Great antigen excess
C. Antigen excess slightly more than equivalence
D. Great antibody avidity for antigen
E. Low antibody avidity for antigen
REF. 7, pp. 541, 552

480. The classical complement pathway is activated by which of the following?
A. Soluble immune complexes
B. Aggregated IgG
C. IgM
D. All of the above
E. None of the above
REF. 7, pp. 548-550

481. The alternative complement pathway is activated by all EXCEPT which of the following?
A. Aggregated IgA
B. C3 nephritic factor
C. Secretory IgA
D. Properdin
E. Endotoxin
REF. 7, pp. 548-550

482. Whcih of the following statements is correct?
A. Depletion of serum complement by cobra venom factor prevents serum sickness in the rabbit
B. All mechanisms in experimental anti-GBM nephritis are dependent on complement
C. Antigens in the plasma membrane of beta-hemolytic streptococci are cross-reactive with human GBM
D. Hageman factor does not play a role in immunologically-mediated glomerular disease
E. None of the above
REF. 7, pp. 548-550

483. Which of the following statements are FALSE?
   A. Lymphocytes from patients with poststreptococcal glomerulonephritis are stimulated by streptococcal antigens
   B. Lymphocytes of patients with anti-GBM antibody nephritis are stimulated by solubilized GBM
   C. Lymphocytes of rats with kidney-in-adjuvant (Heyman) nephritis are stimulated by proximal tubular epithelial antigen
   D. None of the above is false
   E. All of the above are false
   REF. 7, p. 552

484. Which of the following is important in the pathogenesis of immunologically mediated glomerular disease?
   A. Type of antigen
   B. Quantity of antibody response
   C. Complement activation
   D. Only A and C
   E. A, B, and C
   REF. 13, p. 330

485. In immunologically-mediated glomerulonephritis, which of the following statements is FALSE?
   A. PMN participation is important
   B. Activity of the RES may modify the immune response
   C. There may be an activation of the coagulation cascade
   D. The human glomerulus lacks a receptor for C3B
   E. Different immunological insults may produce the same histopathology
   REF. 13, pp. 330-331

486. In which of the following conditions is serum C3 LEAST likely to be decreased?
   A. Acute poststreptococcal GN
   B. Berger's disease (IgA nephropathy)
   C. Lupus nephritis
   D. Hepatitis-B-associated nephritis
   E. Shunt nephritis
   REF. 10, p. 1401

487. The clinical presentation of glomerulonephritis could be
A. an acute nephritic syndrome
B. a nephrotic syndrome
C. an acute nephritic syndrome with nephrotic proteinuria
D. persistent asymptomatic proteinuria with or without hematuria
E. all of the above
REF. 13, p. 332

488. Which of the following statements regarding minimal change disease (MCD) is FALSE?
A. History of atopic disorder often present
B. Over 90% of children remit with prednisone
C. Relapses are rare
D. Most relapses occur within the first 3 months
E. Relapses decrease with time
REF. 13, pp. 337-343

489. Regarding MCD, which of the following statements is FALSE?
A. Remissions may occur without treatment
B. Mortality rarely occurs
C. The use of penicillin has not improved mortality
D. Frequent relapsers may respond to cyclophosphamide
E. Glomerular mesangial hypercellularity may be seen
REF. 13, pp. 337-343

490. Regarding neoplasia and MCD, which of the following statements is FALSE
A. The most common neoplasm is Hodgkin's disease
B. The nephrotic syndrome appears many years before the Hodgkin's disease
C. The nephrotic syndrome remits with remission of Hodgkin's disease
D. All of the above are false
E. None of the above is false
REF. 7, p. 771

491. Which of the following associations between glomerular disease and neoplasia is correct?
A. Membranous nephropathy with solid tumors
B. Lipoid nephrosis with Hodgkin's disease
C. Membranoproliferative glomerulonephritis and leukemia
D. Membranous nephropathy and lymphoma
E. All of the above are correct
REF. 7, pp. 770-771

492. In patients with MCD, a plasma factor has been detected that does which of the following?
  A. Decreases dermal vascular permeability in pigs
  B. Abolishes lymphocyte-mediated glomerular epithelial cell injury
  C. Inhibits PHA-induced blastogenesis in lymphocytes
  D. All of the above
  E. None of the above
  REF. 7, p. 552

493. Which of the following features is NOT common to both MCD and focal segmental glomerulosclerosis?
  A. Predominance in males
  B. Reported familial incidence
  C. Proteinuria is highly selective
  D. The nephrotic syndrome is the usual presenting feature
  E. Serum C3 is normal
  REF. 10, pp. 1419-1427, 1431-1436

494. Which of the following statements about MCD is FALSE?
  A. The peak incidence is between the ages of 2 and 4 years
  B. MCD causes about 20% of cases of the nephrotic syndrome in adults
  C. Males predominate by about 2 to 1
  D. Properdin levels are often decreased
  E. Occurrence in siblings has been reported
  REF. 10, pp. 1419-1429

495. Epithelial cell foot process fusion seen on electron microscopy does NOT occur in
  A. toxemia of pregnancy
  B. aminonucleoside nephrosis
  C. lipoid nephrosis
  D. benign nephrosclerosis
  E. diabetic glomerulosclerosis
  REF. 13, pp. 188-189

496. Which of the following features is NOT characteristic of MCD?
  A. Selective proteinuria
  B. Predominance in childhood
  C. Hypertension
  D. Sudden onset
  E. Good outcome
  REF. 13, pp. 338-343

497. In MCD, which one of the following statements is correct?
A. Corticosteroids alway cause a remission
B. Unless cyclophosphamide is used, relapses will always recur
C. 60% of patients will remit in 2 years without treatment
D. Only 20% will have a spontaneous remission at 2 years
E. Frequent steroid-responsive relapsers progress to renal failure
REF. 13, p. 339

498. Mortality in MCD is primarily due to
A. renal failure
B. infection
C. prednisone
D. adrenal failure after cessation of prednisone
E. thromboembolism
REF. 13, p. 340

499. Given time, MCD may develop
A. membranous change
B. membranoproliferative change
C. crescent formation
D. focal and segmental sclerosing lesions
E. none of the above
REF. 13, p. 342

500. Focal and segmental sclerosis can be seen in which of the following?
A. Hemolytic uremic syndrome
B. Henoch-Schönlein purpura
C. Drug addicts
D. Bacterial endocarditis
E. All of the above
REF. 7, p. 565

501. Which of the following statements about focal and segmental glomerulosclerosis (FSG) is FALSE?
A. Fusion of epithelial cell foot processes
B. The disease is usually progressive
C. Never responds to prednisone
D. Sometimes seen in late biopsies of minimal change disease
E. The nephrotic syndrome is very common
REF. 13, pp. 346-349

502. Which of the following is associated with FGS?
A. Lupus nephritis
B. Reflux nephropathy
C. Scarring stage of focal segmental proliferative glomerulonephritis
D. Massive obesity
E. All of the above
REF. 10, p. 1433

503. Which of the following statements about membranous glomerulonephritis (MGN) is FALSE?
A. Granular immunofluorescence may be seen even when light microscopy is normal
B. Glomerular immune deposits may disappear with clinical remission
C. MGN may be the sole presentation of SLE
D. The deposits are always subepithelial (epimembranous), never intramembranous
E. None of the above is false
REF. 7, pp. 561-562

504. Regarding MGN and neoplasia, which of the following statements is FALSE?
A. Carcinoma of the lung is the most common association
B. The nephrotic syndrome may appear as long as a year before the neoplasia
C. The prognosis for the nephrotic syndrome is always good
D. Tumor antigens have been identified in the glomerular immune deposits
E. MGN may also be seen with lymphoma
REF. 7, p. 771

505. Which of the following neoplasms have been reported with MGN?
A. Lung
B. Colon
C. Kidney
D. Stomach
E. All of the above
REF. 7, p. 771

506. Subepithelial electron-dense deposits are most likely to occur in
A. lipoid nephrosis
B. diabetic glomerulosclerosis
C. amyloidosis
D. penicillamine
E. renal tuberculosis
REF. 10, p. 1437

507. Which of the following features is NOT seen in idiopathic MGN?
A. Most patients are over 40 when first seen
B. Males predominate
C. Onset is insidious
D. C3 and other complement components are generally normal
E. Gross hematuria is common
REF. 10, pp. 1436-1443

508. Membranous glomerulonephritis
A. usually presents with gross hematuria
B. is often associated with Hodgkin's disease
C. never causes chronic renal failure
D. may be associated with renal vein thrombosis
E. very often shows subendothelial electron-dense deposits
REF. 10, pp. 1036-1042

509. Which of the following is NOT a usual presenting feature of MGN?
A. Proteinuria insufficient to produce edema
B. Microscopic hematuria
C. Normal serum complement
D. Nonselective proteinuria
E. Hypertension
REF. 13, p. 344

510. Subepithelial electron-dense humps could be seen in all EXCEPT which of the following?
A. Secondary syphilis
B. SBE
C. Focal glomerulosclerosis
D. Idiopathic MPGN
E. Henoch-Schönlein purpura
REF. 10, p. 1380

511. Acute glomerulonephritis may follow which of the following infections?
A. Typhoid fever
B. Chicken pox
C. Mononucleosis
D. Echo virus infection
E. All of the above
REF. 10, p. 1384

512. In acute poststreptococcal glomerulonephritis (APSGN)
A. ASO titer rises sharply after impetigo
B. anti-DNAase-B titer rises markedly after pharyngitis
C. the classical pathway of complement activation is exclusively involved
D. focal segmental proliferative lesions are characteristic
E. subepithelial electron-dense humps are not pathognomonic
REF. 10, pp. 1373-1385

513. In acute poststreptococcal glomerulonephritis
A. streptococcal pharyngitis or impetigo is always reported by patients
B. males predominate
C. the most common presentation is the nephrotic syndrome
D. the magnitude of rise of ASO titer correlates well with the severity and outcome of the disease
E. none of the above is true
REF. 10, pp. 1373-1385

514. Which of the following statements is FALSE regarding APSGN?
A. Mesangial accentuation may persist for months after clinical recovery
B. Most children recover fully
C. Perhaps a higher percentage of affected adults progress to chronic glomerulonephritis than children
D. Elderly patients do poorly
E. Patients with more than 50% of glomeruli involved by crescents respond promptly to prednisone, cyclophosphamide and plasmapheresis
REF. 10, pp. 1373-1385

515. An acute nephritic syndrome is NOT seen in which of the following?
A. Essential mixed cryoglobulinemia
B. Guillain-Barre-syndrome
C. Acute porphyria
D. After irradiation of solid tumors
E. Coxsackie viral infections
REF. 10, pp. 1384-1385, 1524

516. Which of the following manifestations is LEAST correct in APSGN?
A. Hypertension is unusual at onset
B. Encephalopathy is most common in children
C. Atypical manifestations are more common in the elderly
D. Circulatory congestion may dominate the clinical picture
E. The above results from renal salt and water retention
REF. 10, p. 1375

517. Prognostically, the most unfavorable feature of poststreptococcal glomerulonephritis is
A. severe oliguria
B. hypertension
C. pulmonary edema
D. proteinuria
E. very low serum complement
REF. 10, p. 1384

518. The drug of choice for hypertension developing during acute glomerulonephritis is
A. propranolol
B. oral diuretic
C. methyldopa
D. clonidine
E. hydralazine
REF. 10, p. 1387

519. Regarding resolving APSGN, which of the following statements is FALSE?
A. The electron-dense "humps" usually resolve by 6 weeks
B. Mesangial hypercellularity resolves completely by 8 weeks
C. A little microscopical hematuria and proteinuria may persist for 2 years after clinical recovery
D. ASO returns slowly to normal in several months
E. A very high rate of clinical resolution has been observed in epidemics
REF. 10, pp. 1373-1384

520. In membranoproliferative glomerulonephritis (MPGN), which of the following statements is FALSE?
   A. The double contour (tram track) appearance of glomerular capillary loops is caused by circumferential mesangial interposition
   B. Type I MPGN may show prominent subendothelial deposits
   C. Type II MPGN shows electron-dense transformation of the GBM
   D. Glomerular crescents are very common
   E. Subepithelial "humps" may be seen
   REF. 10, p. 1447

521. Which of the following conditions causes a light microscopical picture resembling MPGN?
   A. Hepatitis B
   B. Allograft glomerulopathy
   C. Mixed cryoglobulinemia
   D. None of the above
   E. All of the above
   REF. 10, p. 1443

522. Which of the following statements about MPGN is FALSE?
   A. The majority of patients will have low serum C3 at initial study
   B. Most patients having C3 NeF in the serum have the type II disease
   C. Serum C3 and C3 NeF levels fluctuate irrespective of disease activity
   D. Serum C1q and C4 are always depressed in type II disease
   E. There is increased catabolism and decreased synthesis of C3
   REF. 10, p. 1445

523. In MPGN, which of the following statements is FALSE?
   A. C3 cleaving factors are not found in other glomerular diseases
   B. There is a particular B-cell antigen in type I MPGN
   C. HLA-B7 is associated with type II MPGN
   D. Serum properdin is normal or decreased
   E. Immune complexes may be detected in type I disease
   REF. 10, p. 1445

524. Which of the following conditions have been reported with MPGN?
   A. C1 inhibitor deficiency
   B. C3 NeF in the serum
   C. C2 deficiency
   D. All of the above
   E. None of the above
   REF. 7, p. 551

525. All of the following diseases may produce a light microscopic picture resembling mesangiocapillary glomerulonephritis EXCEPT
   A. systemic lupus erythematosus
   B. scleroderma
   C. Henoch-Schönlein purpura
   D. poststreptococcal glomerulonephritis
   E. sickle-cell anemia
   REF. 10, p. 1443

526. In reference to anti-GBM antibody GN, which of the following statements is FALSE?
   A. Goodpasture's syndrome refers to anti-GBM antibody nephritis with pulmonary hemorrhage
   B. Pathologically it is usually necrotizing and crescentic and, clinically, rapidly progressive to renal failure
   C. Prednisone, cytoxan, and plasmapheresis will arrest renal disease even if azotemia is far advanced
   D. There is usually linear GBM fluorescence with IgG and C3
   E. Linear fluorescence in the glomerulus does not necessarily indicate anti-GBM GN
   REF. 10, pp. 1386-1394

527. Which is FALSE regarding crescentic GN?
   A. It may be mediated by antibodies to the GBM
   B. It may be mediated by immune complexes
   C. Immunoflourescence may be negative
   D. It may be superimposed on another form of glomerulonephritis
   E. Clinically, a rapidly progressive course to renal failure is rare
   REF. 10, pp. 1385-1394

528. Which of the following statements does NOT apply to anti-GBM antibody nephritis without pulmonary hemorrhage?
A. The usual patient is a young or middle-aged male
B. A preceding flu-like illness may be seen
C. The majority of cases present with sudden anuria
D. Rheumatoid arthritis-like features may be seen
E. Hypertension is typically mild
REF. 10, p. 1388

529. Clinically, rapidly progressive glomerulonephritis does NOT occur in which of the following?
A. SLE
B. Cryoglobulinemia
C. Bacterial endocarditis
D. Lipoid nephrosis
E. Henoch-Schönlein purpura
REF. 10, p. 1387

530. In the treatment of anti-GBM antibody nephritis, which of the following has an established benefit?
A. Heparin
B. Coumadin
C. Dipyridamole
D. Pulse therapy with methyl prednisone
E. None of the above
REF. 10, p. 1391

531. In anti-GBM antibody GN, which of the following statements is correct?
A. Spontaneous recovery is frequent
B. Serum titer of anti-GBM antibody directly correlates with severity and outcome of disease
C. Recurrence rate in transplants is 10-30%
D. Delaying transplantation until serum anti-GBM antibody titer declines does not decrease disease recurrence rate
E. Bilateral nephrectomy prior to transplantation definitely decreases recurrence rate
REF. 10, p. 1391

532. In anti-GBM antibody nephritis, which of the following is NOT a poor prognostic feature?
   A. Over 80% of glomeruli involved by circumferential crescents
   B. Gross hematuria
   C. Severe interstitial fibrosis and tubular atrophy
   D. Glomerular sclerosis and fibrotic crescents
   E. Oliguria
   REF. 10, pp. 1390-1391

533. In Goodpasture's syndrome which statement is FALSE?
   A. It is synonymous with anti-GBM antibody GN with pulmonary hemorrhage
   B. The pulmonary hemorrhage always ceases after bilateral nephrectomy
   C. Anti-GBM antibodies are cross-reactive with alveolar membranes
   D. Pulmonary hemorrhage may be clinically overlooked
   E. Aggressive plasma exchange therapy may arrest the pulmonary hemorrhage
   REF. 10, pp. 1513-1518

534. Pulmonary hemorrhage may be seen in which of the following?
   A. SLE
   B. Henoch-Schönlein purpura
   C. Hypersensitivity angiitis
   D. Legionnaires' disease
   E. All of the above
   REF. 10, p. 1515

535. In Berger's disease (IgA nephropathy) which of the following statements is FALSE?
   A. The most common clinical presentation is asymptomatic microscopic hematuria
   B. Males predominate
   C. Very few blacks are affected
   D. High association with upper respiratory infections
   E. Dysuria often leads to unnecessary urological investigations
   REF. 10, p. 1400

536. In Berger's disease which of the following statements is FALSE?
   A. The nephrotic syndrome is common
   B. Occurrence in siblings and identical twins has been reported
   C. Cyclic neutropenia may be seen
   D. Pulmonary hemosiderosis has been reported
   E. The majority of patients show a slow decrease in the GFR
   REF. 10, pp. 1400-1401

537. Which of the following statements is correct in regard to Berger's disease?
   A. The most common histopathological lesion is a diffuse mesangial hypercellularity
   B. IgA mesangial deposits are seen even in glomeruli normal by light microscopy
   C. A rapidly progressive GN with crescents is very common
   D. Mesangial IgA fluorescence is pathognomonic of IgA nephropathy
   E. All of the above
   REF. 10, pp. 1400-1401

538. In Berger's disease which of the following statements is FALSE?
   A. Serum IgA is increased
   B. Serum C3 is decreased, but C4 is normal
   C. C3 fragments may be increased
   D. A cold reactive antibody to organ-specific nuclear antigen may be found
   E. Circulating IgA-containing immune complexes may be demonstrated
   REF. 10, p. 1401

539. Mesangial IgA deposits are NOT seen in
   A. healthy adults
   B. alcoholic cirrhosis
   C. Henoch-Schönlein purpura
   D. SLE
   E. amyloidosis
   REF. 10, p. 1401

540. Which of the following is NOT common to both Berger's disease and Henoch-Schönlein purpura?
A. Mesangial IgA
B. IgA, C3, properdin, and fibrin in dermal capillaries
C. Leukocytoclastic angiitis
D. Focal-segmental proliferative GN
E. Normal serum C3
REF. 10, p. 1401

541. Which of the following will almost certainly suggest the presence of mesangial IgA?
A. High serum IgA
B. Recurrent hematuria
C. IgA and C3 in dermal capillaries
D. IgG and IgM in dermal capillaries
E. A, B, and C
REF. 10, pp. 1405-1406

542. Recurrent hematuria could be seen in which of the following?
A. Alport's syndrome
B. Fabry's disease
C. Thin GBM
D. All of the above
E. A and C only
REF. 10, pp. 1405-1406

543. Which of the following is NOT associated with the loin pain-hematuria syndrome?
A. Abnormalities of intrarenal vessels
B. Young females
C. Contraceptive steroids
D. Mesangial IgA
E. C3 in renal vessels
REF. 110, pp. 1405-1406

544. Focal segmental glomerulonephritis is seen in all EXCEPT which of the following?
A. SLE
B. Acute poststreptococcal GN
C. Polyarteritis nodosa
D. Henoch-Schönlein purpura
E. Bacterial endocarditis
REF. 13, p. 363

545. Which of the following glomerular diseases recurs in the transplanted kidney?
A. FGS
B. MPGN
C. Anti-GBM antibody GN
D. Berger's disease
E. All of the above
REF. 10, pp. 1373-1457

546. A 45-year-old man with long-standing rheumatoid arthritis develops nephrotic edema; there are red cells in the urine and the 2-hour postprandial blood glucose level is 200 mg%. After a 6-week course of high-dose steroid therapy, the proteinuria is unchanged. Which of the following changes is LEAST likely?
A. Amyloidosis
B. Chronic membranous nephropathy
C. Normal glomeruli on light microscopy
D. Renal vein thrombosis
E. Nodular glomerulosclerosis
REF. 13, pp. 337-343

547. Cyclophosphamide therapy in the nephrotic syndrome has been of proven value in
A. the remission of membranous glomerulonephritis
B. relapsing steroid-sensitive nephrotic syndrome due to the minimal lesion type in childhood
C. proliferative glomerulonephritis
D. the nephrotic syndrome of infancy
E. hereditary nephritis
REF. 13, pp. 341-342

548. Regarding the 5- and 10-year survival rates of glomerulonephritis, which statement is FALSE?

	% Survival	
	5-year	10-year
A. Minimal change	98	97
B. FGS	71	48
C. MGN	40	20
D. MPGN type I	84	64
E. Crescentic GN 80% crescents)	8	3

REF. 13, p. 370

549. Regarding the prognosis of GN, which is a correct statement?
   A. Type II MPGN better than type I MPGN
   B. Idiopathic mesangial proliferative GN worse than APSGN
   C. Focal segmental sclerosis (FGS) in a late biopsy in a steroid-responsive nephrotic syndrome better than FGS in an early biopsy
   D. APSGN with 50% crescents worse than idiopathic anti-GBM antibody GN with 50% crescents
   E. Global glomerulosclerosis in a long-standing steroid-responsive nephrotic syndrome worse than FGS in the same setting

   REF. 13, pp. 346–348, 370

DIRECTIONS: Each group of questions below consists of lettered headings followed by a list of numbered words or statements. For each numbered word or statement, select the one lettered heading that is most closely associated with it. Each lettered heading may be selected once, more than once, or not at all.

A. "One shot" serum sickness in the rabbit
B. Nephritis in NZB/NZW female hybrid mice
C. Heteronephrotoxic serum nephritis (Masugi)
D. Kidney-in-adjuvant nephritis (Heymann)

REF. 7, pp. 541-566

550. Goodpasture's syndrome
551. APSGN
552. MGN
553. Lupus nephritis
554. Idiopathic anti-GBM antibody nephritis

A. Granular glomerular immunofluorescence for immunoglobulins and/or complement
B. Linear GBM immunofluorescence for IgG
C. Neither A nor B

555. MCD
556. APSGN
557. FGS
558. MPGN
559. MGN
560. Goodpasture's syndrome
561. Berger's disease
REF. 7, pp. 553-566

A. C3b
B. C42
C. C7, 8, 9
D. C3a
E. C3bBb

562. C3 converting enzyme(s) for classical complement pathway
563. C3 converting enzyme(s) for alternative complement pathway
564. Causes immune adherence
565. Causes anaphylaxis
566. Causes PMN chemotaxis
567. Lyses cell membranes
REF. 7, pp. 548-549

A. Anti-GBM antibody-mediated pathogenesis
B. Probable immune complex pathogenesis
C. Possible immune complex pathogenesis
D. Nonimmune pathogenesis

568. APSGN
569. Berger's disease
570. Goodpasture's syndrome
571. Polycystic renal disease
572. Minimal change
573. GN associated with SBE
574. MPGN
575. Fabry's disease
REF. 7, p. 553

A. Mainly classical complement pathway activation
B. Mainly alternative pathway activation
C. Both pathways are involved
D. Complement-independent

576. Berger's disease
577. Lupus nephritis
578. GN with SBE
579. APSGN
580. MPGN type I
581. MPGN type II (dense deposit disease)
REF. 7, pp. 550, 553-566

A. Partial lipodystrophy
B. Intravenous drug abuse
C. Endocapillary GN that heals in the great majority of children
D. Better than 90% response rate to prednisone
E. May be the earliest manifestation of a tumor
F. Very rapid progression to renal failure
G. Recurrent macroscopical hematuria

582. Lipoid nephrosis
583. FGS
584. MGN
585. APSGN
586. Focal GN
587. MPGN
588. Anti-GBM antibody GN
REF. 10, pp. 1373-1457

A. Dense transformation of the GBM giving it an "Italian sausage" appearance
B. GBM "spikes" on silver stain
C. Necrotizing GN with circumferential glomerular crescents
D. May be missed if juxtamedullary glomeruli are not sampled
E. "Tram track" or double contour appearance on PAS and silver stains
F. Normal glomeruli on light microscopy
G. Resolving stage may simulate mesangial PGN

589. MCD
590. FGS
591. MGN
592. APSGN
593. MPGN type I
594. MPGN type II
595. Anti-GBM GN
REF. 10, pp. 1373-1457

A. Dense deposits within the GBM
B. Subepithelial electron-dense "humps"
C. Linear staining for IgG along GBM
D. Subepithelial deposits on EM may be seen in early cases when glomeruli are normal on light microscopy
E. Uniform epithelial cell foot process fusion
F. Circumferential mesangial extension into GBM with or without subendothelial deposits

596. MCD
597. MGN
598. APSGN
599. MPGN type I
600. MPGN type II
601. Anti-GBM GN
REF. 10, pp. 1373-1457

6. URINARY TRACT INFECTION AND INTERSTITIAL NEPHRITIS

DIRECTIONS: Each of the questions or incomplete statements below is followed by a list of suggested answers or completions. Select the one that is best in each case.

---

602. Which is NOT true of urinary tract infections (UTI)?
    A. Pregnant women have optimal urinary pH for bacterial growth
    B. Most cases of E. coli pyelonephritis are due to hematogenous spread
    C. Urethral and introital carriage of E. coli is among women with recurrent UTI
    D. Lower pH inhibits bacterial growth
    E. Higher osmolality inhibits bacterial growth
    REF. 12, p. 1573

603. Which of the following is true of UTI?
    A. Majority of episodes are caused by proteus
    B. Renal calculi are common with E. coli infections
    C. Staphylococcus aureus infection commonly results from chronic catheterization
    D. Incidence of proteus UTI is higher among boys than girls (ages 1 through 12)
    E. Systemic antifungal agents are always needed to treat candidal cystitis
    REF. 12, p. 1574

604. Which is an INCORRECT statement regarding staphylococcal UTI?
    A. Occurs with increased frequency in patients with diabetes mellitus
    B. Perinephric abscess accounts for most of the staph UTI
    C. Absence of bacteriuria does not necessarily rule out perinephric abscess

D. Parenchymal abscesses may result from staph aureus endocarditis
E. Coagulase-negative staphylococci can cause significant UTI
REF. 12, p. 1574-1575

605. Regarding hematogenous UTI, which one is true?
A. Pyelonephritis is very common in septicemia
B. Obstruction to urine flow predisposes to E. coli UTI
C. E. coli UTI is generally due to hematogenous spread
D. Hematogenous spread accounts for over half of the cases of UTI
E. Kidneys are very susceptible to hematogenous UTI
REF. 12, p. 1576-1577

606. Which one is an INCORRECT statement regarding UTI in women?
A. Rate of bacteriuria in nuns increases with age like general population
B. Shorter urethra has protective effect
C. Incidence of bacteriuria increases by urethral milking
D. Sexual intercourse contributes to UTI
E. Rise in rate of bacteriuria with age may not be solely related to sexual activity
REF. 12, p. 1578

607. Which one is NOT true regarding vesicoureteral reflux (VUR) in children?
A. Rarely seen in black children
B. More common in females
C. Can be an inherited disorder
D. Can be caused by infection
E. Can be ameliorated by antibiotics in many cases
REF. 12, pp. 1580-1582

608. Regarding intrarenal reflux, which one is true?
A. Bears no relationship to pyelonephritis
B. Never seen in children without renal disease
C. Tends to occur in the middle portions
D. Tends to occur in upper and lower poles
E. Renal scarring is a late phenomenon
REF. 12, pp. 1884-1886

609. Which one is a FALSE statement regarding bacteriuria in childhood?
A. Most of the recurrences involve relapse with the same organism

B. It can cause renal damage when associated with VUR or anatomic abnormality
C. Intermittent therapy does not prevent renal damage
D. Continuous low-dose prophylaxis offers good protection against renal damage
E. At the initial IVP, renal scarring may be seen in 13% of cases

REF. 12, pp. 1601-1603

610. Which of the following is true regarding bacteriuria during pregnancy?
A. Rarely leads to overt pyelonephritis
B. Does not predispose patients to toxemia
C. Long-term outcome is same as nonbacteriuric women
D. Does not need active treatment
E. Is usually due to S. aureus

REF. 12, pp. 1604-1605

611. Which of the following is true of antibody-coated bacteria in UTI?
A. It may be more indicative of invasive infection of uroepithelium than of the exact site of infection
B. There is poor correlation between antibody-coating and relapse
C. Lack of antibody-coating correlates poorly with satisfactory response
D. False-positive results are rare
E. False-negative results are rare

REF. 12, pp. 1610-1611

DIRECTIONS: The group of questions below consists of lettered headings followed by a list of numbered words or statements. For each numbered word or statement, select the one that is most closely associated with it. Each lettered heading may be selected once, more than once, or not at all.

Match the following numbered statements with the lettered ones. Each lettered statement to be used only once.

A. Can cause peripheral neuropathy and precipitate hemolysis in G-6-PD-deficiency patients
B. Can cause kernicterus in infant if used in third trimester or in neonates
C. Best suited for prostatitis

D. Recommended for serratia and pseudomonas UTI
E. Must be avoided during pregnancy for the fear of hepatic dysfunction in mother and dental dysplasia in fetus

612. Trimethoprim-sulfamethoxazole
613. Sulfonamides
614. Tetracyclines
615. Nitrofurantoins
616. Aminoglycosides

REF. 12, pp. 1612-1613

DIRECTIONS: Each of the questions or incomplete statements below is followed by a list of suggested answers or completions. Select the one that is best in each case.

---

617. Which one is NOT true regarding catheter-associated UTI?

A. Most common nosocomial infection
B. Bladder irrigation is helpful
C. Systemic amphotericin-B is always indicated for candida infection
D. No treatment may be needed for infections due to short term catheterization
E. Oral 5-fluorocytosine is effective for candida infection

REF. 12, pp. 1616-1617

618. Which of the following is most helpful in pathologically distinguishing chronic pyelonephritis from chronic glomerulonephritis?

A. Polymorphs in the tubules
B. Tubular dilatation
C. Glomerular sclerosis
D. Inflammation and fibrosis of the calyces
E. Tubular atrophy

REF. 3, p. 1329

619. Which of the following is more often a feature of chronic interstitial nephritis than of chronic glomerulonephritis?

A. Proteinuria
B. Low GFR
C. Low renal blood flow
D. Hyperchloremic acidosis
E. Hypochromic microcytic anemia

REF. 2, p. 1654

620. All of the following are true about xanthogranulomatous pyelonephritis EXCEPT
A. there is profound weight loss
B. E. coli is the most common organism
C. lucent areas are seen on nephrotomography
D. it is associated with staghorn calculi
E. radiologically it may mimic a tumor
REF. 3, p. 1381

621. Which of the following cancers is associated with excessive analgesic intake?
A. Gastric carcinoma
B. Hypernephroma
C. Renal pelvis cancer
D. Cancer of the prostate
E. Cancer of the bladder
REF. 3, p. 1237

622. Acute tubulointerstitial nephritis may in part be characterized by all of the following EXCEPT
A. a hypersensitive reaction involving tubules and interstitial tissue rather than glomeruli
B. most reports have implicated sulfonomides, methicillin, or large doses of penicillin
C. arteritis is not a feature but lesions are characterized by irregular interstitial accumulation of leukocytes containing many mononuclear cells
D. hematuria with mild to moderate proteinuria
E. abnormally low BUN
REF. 2, p. 1660

623. Which of the following is LEAST compatible with the diagnosis of interstitial nephritis?
A. Analgesic abuse
B. Vesicoureteric reflux
C. Secondary syphilis
D. Sarcoidosis
E. Amyloidosis
REF. 1, p. 542

624. Which of the following is contraindicated in hyperuricemia?
A. Ammonium chloride
B. Sodium bicarbonate
C. Penicillin
D. Acetozolamide
E. Calcium salts
REF. 1, p. 548

625. Which of the following causes of papillary necrosis usually shows interstitial sclerosis?
A. Ureteral obstruction
B. Diabetes mellitus
C. Analgesic abuse
D. Acute pyelonephritis
E. Amyloidosis
REF. 3, p. 1232

626. Which of the following is characteristic of papillary necrosis due to analgesic abuse?
A. Unequal kidney size
B. Hypertrophied Bertini columns
C. The scars are polar in distribution
D. Dilated calyx
E. All in the same stage of sloughing
REF. 3, p. 1232

627. Which abnormality of the urinary sediment is most compatible with analgesic nephropathy?
A. Red cell casts
B. Oval fat bodies
C. Sterile pyuria
D. Phenacetin crystals
E. Pigmented hyaline casts
REF. 7, p. 825

628. Balkan nephritis
A. is rare in children
B. occurs after living 5 to 10 years in endemic villages
C. occurs in mountaintop villages
D. is not associated with urinary tumors
E. is mainly a glomerular lesion
REF. 3, p. 1173

629. Which of the following does NOT cause renal disease?
A. Penicillin
B. Gentamicin
C. Erythromycin
D. Sulfonamides
E. Cephalothin
REF. 10, p. 2049

7. METABOLIC, CALCULOUS, AND OBSTRUCTIVE DISEASE

DIRECTIONS: Each of the questions or incomplete statements below is followed by five suggested answers or completions. Select the one that is best in each case.

A. Metabolic Disease

630. Increased plasma or tissue erythropoietin-like substances may be found in all of the following EXCEPT
    A. hypernephroma
    B. cerebellar hemangioma
    C. hepatoma
    D. solitary renal cyst
    E. carcinoma of stomach
    REF. 7, p. 286

631. Aminoaciduria, glycosuria, phosphaturia, and severe osteomalacia are classically seen with
    A. methoxyflurane
    B. cadmium
    C. gold
    D. ammoniated mercury
    E. aluminum
    REF. 7, p. 1442

632. Which feature is absent in cadmium nephropathy?
    A. Aminoaciduria
    B. Renal glycosuria
    C. Albuminuria
    D. Low molecular weight proteinuria
    E. Porphyrinuria
    REF. 1, p. 556

633. A 50-year-old farmer who was exposed to pesticide and disinfectant was admitted with a history of nausea, vomiting, metallic taste, and diarrhea. His BUN was 150 mg/100 ml; 24-hour urine output was 300 ml. Urinalysis showed proteinuria, RBC, and epithelial casts. Which of the following would be the treatment of choice?
A. Monitor fluid and electrolyte balance and administer fluids and electrolytes accordingly
B. High dose of costicosteroids
C. Inject dimercaprol (BAL) 3 mg/kg/24 hr
D. Use of gastric lavage
E. Inject dimercaprol (BAL) 3 mg/kg followed by hemodialysis
REF. 1, p. 556

634. Urinary acidification may be of value in the treatment of overdosage of
A. salicylic acid
B. fenfluramine
C. nalidixic acid
D. nitrofurantoin
E. phenylbutazone
REF. 10, p. 2662

635. The concentrating defect in hypokalemic nephropathy is due to
A. diminished GFR
B. increased proximal Na reabsorption
C. diminished Na reabsorption in the loop of Henle
D. insensitivity to ADH
E. damaged distal convoluted tubule
REF. 5, p. 507

636. In man the main histologic abnormality in hypokalemic nephropathy is
A. proximal tubule vacuolation
B. distal tubule vacuolation
C. obstruction of collecting ducts
D. interstitial infiltration
E. interstitial calcification
REF. 5, p. 508

637. Which of the following is LEAST likely to be associated with hypokalemic nephropathy?
   A. Abnormal excretion of PAH and phenolsulfonphthalein
   B. Serum creatinine level of 0.9 mg/100 ml
   C. Impaired concentrating ability
   D. Impaired diluting capacity
   E. Tubular proteinuria
   REF. 1, p. 561

638. Which of the following is diagnostic of hypokalemia nephropathy?
   A. Lack of concentrating ability after infusion of ADH and a serum K of 2 mEq/L
   B. Loss of diluting capacity and serum K level of 2.5 mEq/L
   C. Serum K of 1.2 mEq/L
   D. Serum K of 3.5 mEq/L and glomerular sclerosis
   E. Serum K of 3.5 mEq/L and renal biopsy showing multiple vacuoles in the renal tubular epithelium
   REF. 1, p. 562

639. Potassium-losing nephritis may be suspected when hypokalemia is
   A. associated with hyperchloremic acidosis
   B. completely responsive to spironolactone
   C. associated with alkalosis
   D. associated with high plasma aldosterone
   E. associated with tubular proteinuria
   REF. 1, p. 562

B. Calculous Disease

640. In hot climates which of the following stones are frequently seen?
   A. Cystine
   B. Calcium oxalate
   C. Uric acid
   D. Magnesium phosphate
   E. Triple phosphate
   REF. 5, p. 1524

641. Which is the most important step of vitamin D metabolism carried out in kidney?
A. 25-hydroxylation of cholecalciferol
B. 1-hydroxylation of 25-hydroxycholecalciferol
C. Production of dihydrotachysterol
D. Both 1 and 25-hydroxylation of cholecalciferol
E. Only ergocalciferol may be converted to 1,25-hydroxycholecalciferol
REF. 13, p. 771

642. Calcification of basal ganglia, subcutaneous deposits of calcium, shortening of metacarpal bones, and mental retardation occur in
A. pseudohypoparathyroidism
B. idiopathic hypoparathyroidism
C. postthyroidectomy hypoparathyroidism
D. hyperparathyroidism
E. pseudohyperparathyroidism
REF. 7, p. 1078

643. Which of the following is true of nephrocalcinosis?
A. Not found in distal renal tubular acidosis
B. Not found in medullary sponge kidney
C. Not found in Fanconi's syndrome
D. Not found in hyperparathyroidism
E. Is present in all of the above
REF. 5, p. 916

644. Which is the most common renal stone?
A. Apatite
B. Magnesium ammonium phosphate
C. Uric acid
D. Cysteine
E. Calcium oxalate with or without calcium phosphate
REF. 2, p. 1673

645. Which of the following is NOT true for calcium stone disease?
A. Chlorothiazide is useful to prevent recurrent stone formation
B. Relative alkalinity of the urine may be a factor in calcium stone disease
C. Predominates in renal tubular acidosis
D. Phosphopeptide inhibitor is lacking in the urine of the calcium stone formers
E. Secondary hypercalciuria is the most common cause of calcium stone
REF. 2, p. 1673

646. Ninety percent of all kidney stones contain
  A. calcium
  B. phosphate
  C. uric acid
  D. oxalate
  E. ammonium
  REF. 7, p. 893

647. Stones are caused by all of the following EXCEPT
  A. phosphaturia
  B. hypercalciuria
  C. hyperoxaluria
  D. hyperuricosuria
  E. cystinuria
  REF. 7, p. 894

648. Hypercalciuria with renal stones may be treated with all of the following to reduce urinary calcium excretion EXCEPT
  A. low-salt diet
  B. thiazide diuretics
  C. low-calcium diet
  D. low-phosphate diet
  E. oral phosphate
  REF. 7, p. 917

649. Which is the drug of choice in idiopathic renal hypercalciuria?
  A. Ascorbic acid
  B. Hydrochlorothiazide
  C. Tinacrynic acid
  D. Cortisone
  E. Cellulose phosphate
  REF. 2, p. 1674

650. Inorganic phosphate therapy lowers serum calcium by
  A. decreasing intestinal absorption of calcium
  B. increasing urinary excretion of calcium
  C. decreasing bone resorption
  D. increasing bone formation
  E. increasing fecal excretion of calcium
  REF. 5, p. 1036

651. In hypercalcemic nephropathy the part of the nephron most likely to have calcium deposition is
A. proximal convoluted tubule
B. efferent arterioles
C. distal convoluted tubule
D. loop of Henle
E. none of the above
REF. 7, p. 1414

652. Vitamin D-resistant rickets is
A. sex-linked recessive inheritance
B. caused by decreased calcium absorption by the gut
C. primarily a tubular defect
D. associated with hyperphosphatemia
E. none of the above
REF. 2, p. 1670

653. What is the incidence of nephrolithiasis in primary hyperparathyroidism?
A. 5%
B. 10%
C. 25%
D. 50%
E. 100%
REF. 7, p. 1416

654. In hypercalcemia due to causes other than hyperparathyroidism there usually is all of the following EXCEPT
A. increased ammonia excretion
B. low urine pH
C. raised plasma bicarbonate
D. hyperchloremia
E. none of the above is found
REF. 7, p. 1418

655. In which of the following is increased absorption of calcium NOT the cause of the hypercalcemia?
A. Sarcoidosis
B. Idiopathic hypercalcemia
C. Vitamin D intoxication
D. Multiple myeloma
E. None of the above
REF. 3, p. 1615

656. Hypercalcemia from vitamin D intoxication is mainly due to
A. increased bone resorption
B. decreased fecal excretion of calcium
C. increased gastrointestinal absorption of calcium
D. diminished renal excretion of calcium
E. diminished glomerular filtration
REF. 5, p. 1022

657. Substances that protect against calcium phosphate stone formation are all of the following EXCEPT
A. citrate
B. magnesium
C. pyrophosphate
D. inhibitor polypeptides
E. alkaline urine
REF. 7, p. 918

658. Which of the following is LEAST characteristic of uric acid stones?
A. Radiopaque calculi
B. Passage of reddish gravel
C. Uric acid crystaluria
D. Gouty arthritis
E. A positive family history
REF. 7, p. 911

659. Oxalate stones are LEAST likely to occur with
A. pentazocine
B. ethylene glycol
C. Crohn's disease
D. methoxyflurane
E. large doses of ascorbic acid
REF. 10, p. 1648

660. Hyperoxaluria occurs in all of the following conditions EXCEPT
A. ethylene glycol poisoning
B. excessive pyridoxine intake
C. high intake of oxalate in the diet
D. primary oxaluria
E. inflammatory bowel disease
REF. 7, p. 907

661. Magnesium ammonium phosphate stones are found in association with
A. high magnesium intake
B. high ammonium intake
C. high phosphate intake
D. infection with urea-splitting organisms
E. prolonged excessive use of antacid
REF. 7, p. 921

662. Which of the following statements about cystine stone disease is NOT correct?
A. It is rare and inherited as autosomal recessive character
B. It is associated with the excretion of ornithine, arginine, and lysine
C. There is usually an associated transport defect in the gastrointestinal tract
D. It is usually unilateral
E. It usually occurs when the urinary cystine excretion exceeds 100 mg/24 hr
REF. 2, p. 511

663. Which of the following renal stones is radiolucent?
A. Calcium oxalate
B. Xanthine
C. Cystine
D. Calcium magnesium
E. Calcium phosphate
REF. 1, p. 586

664. A 30-year-old man presented with recurrent stones and x-ray of the abdomen shows bilateral nephrocalcinosis. Which of the following will be the LEAST likely cause?
A. Hyperparathyroidism
B. Sarcoidosis
C. Oxalosis
D. Renal tubular acidosis
E. Cystinuria
REF. 1, p. 586

665. For effective treatment of potential renal stone formers, in which of the following conditions should the urinary pH ideally be maintained at about 8?
A. Cystinuria
B. Uric acid
C. Oxalosis
D. Idiopathic hypercalciuria
E. None of the above
REF. 1, p. 587

666. Which of the following is NOT true for magnesium-ammonium phosphate stone formation?
A. It usually is associated with urinary tract infection
B. It is the principal constituent of the typical staghorn calculus
C. This stone rarely contains calcium phosphate
D. It is highly radiopaque
E. It usually is associated with an alkaline urine
REF. 2, p. 1675

667. Match:
A. Phosphate stones
B. Ca oxalate stones
C. Uric acid stones
D. Cystine stones

1. Waxy yellow
2. Sharp edges
3. Occur in alkaline urine
4. Small, hard, yellow
REF. 2, p. 1672

668. The most common variety of renal stones is
A. uric acid
B. calcium phosphate
C. mixed calcium oxalate/calcium phosphate
D. struvite
E. calcium oxalate
REF. 12, p. 1951

669. Majority of calcium stones tend to recur within
A. 1-5 years
B. 6-9 years
C. 10-15 years
D. 15-20 years
E. never recur
REF. 12, pp. 1954-1956

670. Pregnant women with renal stones have higher rate of
A. preeclampsia
B. urinary tract infection
C. fetal wastage
D. congenital malformation
E. renal failure
REF. 12, p. 1156

671. Which one of the following is NOT an inhibitor of stone formation?
A. Pyrophosphate
B. Mucopolysaccharide
C. Citrate
D. Uromucoids
E. Glycopeptides
REF. 12, pp. 1960-1961

672. All the following statements about primary hyperparathyroidism are true EXCEPT
A. positive calcium balance due to enhanced intestinal absorption of calcium
B. parathormone stimulates synthesis of 1-25 (OH_2) D_3
C. tendency to form stones depends more on calcium excretion than plasma calcium concentration
D. urinary cyclic AMP is helpful in diagnosis
E. progression of renal disease frequently occurs despite successful parathyroidectomy
REF. 12, pp. 1965-1970

673. Which one of the following is NOT a characteristic of idiopathic hypercalciuria?
A. Autosomal dominant trait
B. Elevated fractional excretion of calcium
C. Positive calcium balance is frequent
D. Rate of occurrence is same in children and adults
E. Negative calcium balance is frequent
REF. 12, pp. 1970-1973

674. Which one may NOT be present in "renal" hypercalciuria?
   A. Elevated urinary cyclic AMP
   B. Elevated 1,25 $(OH)_2$ D_3
   C. Reduction in intestinal calcium absorption during thiazide therapy
   D. Decrease in PTH level on low-calcium diet
   E. Reduction in 1,25 $(OH)_2$ D_3 level during thiazide therapy
   REF. 12, p. 1974

675. Which one is true regarding "absorptive" hypercalciuria?
   A. Thiazide decreases intestinal calcium absorption
   B. Patients are at increased risk for developing parathyroid adenoma
   C. Calcium excretion can be normalized on low-calcium diet
   D. High-fasting urinary cyclic AMP
   E. High-fasting PTH levels
   REF. 12, p. 1974

DIRECTIONS: The group of questions below consists of lettered headings followed by a list of numbered words or statements. For each numbered word or statement, select the one that is most closely associated with it. Each lettered heading may be selected once, more than once, or not at all.

A. Calcium phosphate stones; high urine pH
B. Methoxyflurane
C. Pancreatic insufficiency
D. Increased risk of parathyroid adenoma
E. Low urinary cyclic AMP
F. Adsorbs stone inhibitors

676. Absorptive hypercalciuria
677. Renal hypercalciuria
678. Hyperuricosuria
679. Hyperoxaluria
680. Distal RTA
681. Intestinal hyperoxaluria
   REF. 12, pp. 1970-1992

DIRECTIONS: Each of the questions or incomplete statements below is followed by a list of suggested answers or completions. Select the one that is best in each case.

682. Which one of the following is NOT true of hyperuricosuria?
A. Excessive purine intake
B. Uric acid overproduction
C. Allopurinol effective for recurrent stones
D. Lower urinary pH promotes stone formation
E. Majority have hyperuricemia as well
REF. 12, pp. 1981-1985

683. Which one is NOT associated with hyperoxaluria/oxalate stones?
A. Ethylene glycol poisoning
B. Ileostomy for Crohn's disease
C. Jejunocolic bypass
D. Methoxyflurane
E. Pancreatic insufficiency
REF. 12, p. 1992

684. Which of the following is true of uric acid stones?
A. Allopurinol is always indicated
B. Urine pH is very important in stone formation
C. Uncommon in tropical climate
D. Probenecid is the medical treatment of choice
REF. 12, pp. 1992-1996

685. Regarding magnesium-ammonium-phosphate stones, which one of the following statements is true?
A. Excessive magnesium intake
B. Excessive phosphate intake
C. Excessive use of antacids
D. Infection with urea-splitting organisms
E. Surgical treatment is effective and recurrence is rare
REF. 12, pp. 1998-1999

686. Which of the following is a FALSE statement concerning distal RTA and nephrolithiasis ?
   A. Acquired distal RTA does not cause stone formation
   B. Intestinal calcium absorption is elevated and calcium balance is generally positive
   C. Low urinary citrate level
   D. Fractional reabsorption of calcium is reduced even in presence of elevated PTH levels
   E. Alkali administration can prevent stone formation
   REF. 12, pp. 1986-1987

C. Obstructive Disease

687. Urinary tract infection is most likely to occur when the obstruction is in the
   A. pelvis
   B. upper ureter
   C. ureterovesical junction
   D. lower ureter
   E. urethra
   REF. 7, pp. 1006-1007

688. Total anuria is LEAST likely in
   A. acute tubular necrosis
   B. extracapillary glomerulonephritis
   C. ureteral obstruction
   D. diffuse necrotizing glomerulonephritis
   E. bilateral cortical necrosis
   REF. 7, p. 171

689. Which of the following is NOT found in acute unilateral obstruction of the ureter ?
   A. Urine sodium concentration is lower than the control side
   B. Urine osmolality is higher than the control side
   C. Increased DNA synthesis and cell division occur in the obstructed kidney
   D. Rapid improvement in GFR after release of a 5-day obstruction
   E. Increased urinary Na concentration compared with the control side
   REF. 7, p. 1313

690. Which of the following conditions is most likely to be associated with unilateral hydronephrosis?
A. Polycythemia rubra vera
B. Nephrotic syndrome
C. Macrocytic anemia
D. Microangiopathic hemolytic anemia
E. Erythrocytosis
REF. 7, p. 287

691. Which of the following drugs may cause urinary retention?
A. Reserpine
B. Hydralazine
C. Ephedrine
D. Isoniazid
E. All of the above
REF. 1, p. 68

692. Which of the following does NOT produce obstructive uropathy?
A. Warfarin
B. Methysergide
C. Sulfadiazine
D. Phenacetin
E. Phenytoin
REF. 10, p. 2077

693. Obstructive uropathy from retroperitoneal fibrosis is LEAST likely to be associated with
A. migraine headaches
B. mediastinal fibrosis
C. temporal arteritis
D. Riedel struma
E. Dupuytren contracture
REF. 2, p. 1831

694. A 30-year-old female presented with low back pain and urinary tract infection; IVP showed blunting of the minor calyces with ureteral dilatation. Which of the following may be related to the patient's condition?
A. Vague frontal headaches for 10 years
B. Migrainous headaches for 5 years
C. Use of contraceptive pill for 10 years
D. Use of Pro-Banthine daily for 6 weeks for peptic ulcer
E. History of herpes zoster 2 years ago
REF. 1, p. 1901

695. Renal failure in paraplegics is most closely related to
A. hydronephrosis
B. renal calculus
C. reflux
D. caliectasis
E. none of the above
REF. 3, p. 1283

696. Which of the following is true for reflux in childhood?
A. Patients showing infection should have the ureter implanted surgically
B. Medical treatment is usually hopeless
C. Tendency to reflux gradually increases with age
D. Most of the patients with reflux show permanent renal damage
E. None of the above
REF. 7, p. 1115

697. Which of the following drugs achieve effective concentration in prostatic secretions?
A. Penicillin
B. Sulfonamides
C. Streptomycin
D. Erythromycin
E. None of the above
REF. 2, p. 1655

698. Relative ineffectiveness of antimicrobials in prostatic infection is due to which of the following?
A. Lack of adequate vascular supply
B. Poor penetration due to low pH in this organ
C. Poor penetration due to high pH in this organ
D. Most of the infections are not due to common pathogens of urinary tract infection
E. Rapid development of resistance
REF. 2, p. 1655

699. A 70-year-old man is hospitalized because of uremia. Three years earlier he had a colostomy for cancer of the colon, and postoperatively he had an episode of podagra. Urine output is 1000 ml/24 hr, BUN 120 mg/100 ml, and serum uric acid is 12 mg/100 ml. Which of the following statements is most applicable?
A. The most likely diagnosis is uric acid nephropathy and treatment with allopurinol should be started
B. The patient probably has immune complex disease, and treatment will depend on the carcinoembryonic antigen titer in the blood
C. The high urine output excludes any significant obstructive uropathy
D. The patient probably has bilateral infiltration of the renal parenchyme by cancer cells
E. The obstruction of the ureters may be incomplete
REF. 7, p. 880

700. After release of ureteral obstruction the fractional Na excretion is
A. increased in acute obstruction
B. unchanged in acute obstruction
C. increased in chronic obstruction
D. decreased in chronic obstruction
E. the same in acute and chronic obstruction
REF. 7, p. 887

701. Natriuresis following relief of bilateral obstruction of the urinary tract is the result of all of the following EXCEPT
A. impaired sodium reabsorption in the proximal tubule
B. impaired sodium reabsorption in ascending limb of loop of Henle
C. passive sodium influx back into the tubular fluid
D. osmotic urea diuresis
E. presence of natriuretic hormone
REF. 7, p. 887

702. The major functional abnormality in postobstructive diuresis is
A. diminished concentrating ability of the collecting tubule
B. diminished sodium reabsorption in the loop of Henle
C. diminished sodium reabsorption in the proximal tubule
D. increased renal blood flow
E. none of the above
REF. 7, p. 887

703. In long-standing urinary tract obstruction, when the obstruction is released which of the following is NOT usually present?
A. Hyponatremia
B. Low urinary excretion of sodium
C. Hyposthenuria
D. Osmotic diuresis
E. Excretion of more than 60% of the filtered urea
REF. 1, p. 546

704. Pneumaturia is most common in the
A. elderly male
B. young female
C. patient with indwelling catheter
D. patient with anaerobic urinary tract infection
E. elderly diabetic woman
REF. 1, p. 440

705. Which of the following will suggest the diagnosis of chyluria?
A. Milky urine associated with pyelonephritis
B. Clear urine
C. Nephrotic syndrome
D. Postural milky urine
E. None of the above
REF. 1, p. 1775

706. The major component of chyluria is
A. albumin
B. lecithin
C. fibrinogen
D. triglycerides
E. cholesterol
REF. 1, p. 1775

8. RENAL INVOLVEMENT IN SYSTEMIC DISEASE

DIRECTIONS: Each of the questions or incomplete statements below is followed by five suggested answers or completions. Select the one that is best in each case.

---

707. Which one of the following is NOT seen in the early stages of diabetic nephropathy?
    A. Microalbuminuria
    B. Enlargement of the kidneys
    C. Decreased glomerular filtration rate
    D. Increased filtration fraction
    E. Increased tubular maximal capacity for glucose reabsorption
    REF. 10, p. 1912

708. In diabetic nephropathy
    A. the diffuse lesion correlates poorly with the severity of the disease
    B. the nodules are generally hypercellular and uniform in size
    C. the efferent arterioles are thickened
    D. extramembranous deposits are the rule
    E. the hyaline cap precedes the glomerulosclerosis
    REF. 10, p. 1907

709. The most frequent immunoflourescent finding in glomeruli of diabetic nephropathy is
    A. a granular (lumpy-bumpy) pattern
    B. mesangial deposits
    C. complement deposits
    D. a linear pattern
    E. IgE deposits
    REF. 8, p. 572

710. The vascular lesions of diabetic nephropathy include all of the following EXCEPT
A. nodular glomerulosclerosis
B. arteritis
C. diffuse glomerulosclerosis
D. hyaline cap
E. capsular drop
REF. 7, p. 1199

711. Which one of the following is most likely to hasten the decline of renal function in advanced diabetic nephropathy?
A. Bacteriuria
B. Hypertension
C. Bladder detrusor dysfunction
D. Hyperglycemia
E. Hypoaldosteronism
REF. 11 (5), pp. 142, 171

712. In the presence of diabetic nephropathy and the nephrotic syndrome
A. urinary tract obstruction is best ruled out by intravenous urography
B. hypertension is often present
C. retinopathy is usually absent
D. response to steroids is usually good
E. proteinuria is often selective
REF. 8, p. 571

713. Which of the following has NOT been implicated in inducing SLE?
A. Isoniazid
B. Hydralazine
C. Phenytoin
D. Procainamide
E. Nitrofurantoin
REF. 1, pp. 381, 1856

714. Which of the following is LEAST indicative of active glomerular disease in systemic lupus?
A. High antinuclear antibody titer
B. Antibodies to double-stranded DNA
C. Reduced complement levels
D. Immune complexes in the serum
E. Cryoimmunoglobulinemia
REF. 10, p. 1506

715. Which glomerular lesion is considered to be most specific of systemic lupus erythematosus?
A. Focal necrosis
B. Hematoxylin bodies
C. Wire loop lesions
D. Tubuloreticular arrays
E. Hyaline thrombi
REF. 1, pp. 534-535

716. In considering renal involvement in SLE which of the following statements is INCORRECT?
A. A telescoped urinary sediment is highly suggestive of active nephritis
B. Antibodies to single-stranded DNA occur more frequently with drug-induced lupus
C. Proteinuria per se is an accurate indication of active nephritis
D. C_4 is a better indication of activity than C_3
E. A normal level of antibodies to double-stranded DNA suggests inactive or quiescent renal disease
REF. 10, p. 1495

717. Which of the following forms of lupus nephritis has the WORST prognosis?
A. Mesangial
B. Focal segmental
C. Diffuse proliferative
D. Membranous
E. Interstitial
REF. 1, p. 535

718. In a patient with active lupus erythematosus who has impaired renal function but relatively normal glomeruli on renal biopsy, the finding of interstitial infiltrates and immunoglobulin deposits along the tubular basement membranes is most compatible with
A. analgesic nephropathy
B. hypersensitivity to hydralazine
C. lupus interstitial nephritis
D. furosemide-induced interstitial nephritis
E. hypersensitivity to nonsteroidal anti-inflammatory drugs
REF. 12(10), pp. 138, 170

719. Focal and segmental lupus nephritis
A. is the most severe form of renal involvement
B. causes nephrotic syndrome in 80% of cases
C. often has a linear immunofluorescent pattern
D. generally requires low-dose steroid treatment
E. usually requires intense plasma exchange
REF. 12(3), pp. 269-274

720. Concerning the relationship of systemic lupus erythematosus and pregnancy, which of the following statements is NOT true?
A. The fertility rate of women with lupus is similar to that of normal women
B. During pregnancy about one-half of patients exhibit no change, one-third may become worse (especially during the first trimester), and a few patients improve
C. Most series report a two- to threefold increase in prematurity and spontaneous abortion
D. There is no evidence that steroids given during pregnancy have a teratogenic effect
E. Exacerbations of the disease during the postpartum period are rare
REF. 10, p. 1788

721. Procainamide-induced LE syndrome rarely produces which one of the following features?
A. Antinuclear antibodies
B. Positive direct Coombs test
C. Massive proteinuria
D. Pulmonary infiltrates
E. Arthralgia
REF. 1, p. 1856

722. Which of the following is NOT true for hydralazine-induced LE syndrome?
A. Antibodies to histones are common
B. Renal disease is rare
C. Symptoms usually stop after cessation of the drug
D. Fast-acetylators are more often affected
E. Most cases occur following high doses of the drug
REF. 1, p. 1856

723. Which one of the following is likely to occur in the highest titer in a 40-year-old woman suffering from arthralgias, swelling of the fingers, Raynaud's phenomenon, dysphagia, and mild proteinuria?
   A. Anti-Sm antibody
   B. Antibody to saline-extractable ribonuclear protein antigen
   C. Single-stranded DNA antibody
   D. Double-stranded DNA antibody
   E. Antinuclear antibody
   REF. 1, p. 1860

724. With reference to the genetic basis of systemic lupus erythematosus, which one of the following statements is INCORRECT?
   A. A 63% concordance has been observed in monozygotic twins
   B. In monozygotic twins the clinical manifestations are similar
   C. IgA and complement deficiencies may occur
   D. No HLA predilection has been described
   E. Other connective tissue disorders and autoimmune phenomena occur in about 5% of first degree relatives
   REF. 1, p. 1853

725. On the serologic diagnosis of systemic lupus erythematosus all but which one of the following applies?
   A. Homogenous nuclear fluorescence reflects antibodies to nucleoprotein, usually double-stranded DNA, and is positive in 90% of SLE patients but also in 15-40% of other connective tissue disease
   B. A rim or peripheral pattern can occur in association with antibodies directed against either double- or single-stranded DNA, and thus is less specific
   C. A nucleolar pattern represents antibodies to a nuclear RNA and often occurs in scleroderma
   D. A speckled pattern reflects antibodies to extractable nuclear antigens or Sm antigen
   E. Antibodies to double-stranded DNA are found in 20% of untreated SLE
   REF. 12(3), p. 271

726. In lupus nephritis which one of the following does NOT apply?
A. Glomerular receptors for C_3 may occur
B. Subendothelial deposits tend to resolve with therapy
C. A circulating coagulant has been related to glomerular capillary thrombosis
D. Complement activation tends to be through the alternate pathway
E. Associated thrombotic phenomenon may occur
REF. 11(6), p. 14

727. Pulmonary hemorrhage with nephritis is LEAST likely in
A. SLE
B. scleroderma
C. Henoch-Schönlein syndrome
D. Goodpasture's syndrome
E. polyarteritis nodosa
REF. 1, p. 1858

728. Which of the following is LEAST likely in a patient with hematuria, hemoptysis, proteinuria, low complement, and granular immunofluorescence on renal biopsy?
A. Circulating immune-complexes and cryoglobulinemia
B. Elevated serum IgA levels
C. Antiglomerular basement membrane antibodies
D. Fever, arthritis, and mononeuritis multiplex
E. Focal and segmental necrotizing glomerular lesions
REF. 8, p. 566

729. In patients with Goodpasture's syndrome, which of the following statements is LEAST appropriate?
A. Diffuse crescentic or focal segmental varieties of glomerulonephritis are frequently observed
B. Pulmonary hemorrhage may lead to iron deficiency and hemosiderin-filled macrophages may be found in the sputum
C. Plasmapheresis associated with cytotoxic drugs and corticosteroids may produce substantial improvement
D. Nephrectomy controls severe pulmonary bleeding and should be considered early
E. Renal transplantation is contraindicated when circulating antiglomerular basement membrane antibody is detectable
REF. 8, p. 567

730. In Goodpasture's syndrome all of the following are characteristic EXCEPT
A. massive proteinuria and the nephrotic syndrome
B. absent circulating immune complexes and cryoglobulins
C. progressive renal failure
D. pulmonary infiltrates
E. glomerular crescents
REF. 10, p. 1515

731. A woman with extensive scleroderma, treated for some time with naproxen and penicillamine, abruptly develops severe hypertension and becomes anuric. A renal biopsy, would most likely show
A. severe extracapillary glomerulonephritis
B. severe interstitial inflammation
C. thickening of interlobular arteries and fibrinoid necrosis of arterioles
D. severe endothelial proliferation
E. sclerosis of 80% of glomeruli
REF. 10, pp. 1680-1682

732. In the patient described above, which one of the following is NOT likely to be present?
A. Hypocomplementemia
B. Hyperreninemia
C. A speckled fluorescent ANA pattern
D. Microangiopathic hemolytic anemia
E. Antibodies to single-stranded DNA
REF. 8, p. 561

733. In considering the therapy of this patient, which of the following is true?
A. Hypertension should not be treated because it will worsen renal function
B. Treatment with prednisone may be life-saving
C. Early nephrectomy and renal transplantation should be considered
D. Recovery of renal function is unlikely but has been reported
E. The administration of captopril is contraindicated
REF. 11(4), pp. 268-269

734. In considering renal involvement in infective endocarditis which of the following manifestations is unusual?
A. Gross hematuria
B. Nephrotic syndrome
C. Acute nephritis syndrome with azotemia
D. Rapidly progressive renal failure
E. Presence of cryoimmunoglobulins
REF. 10, p. 1536

735. Amyloidosis of the kidney has been associated with all of the following EXCEPT
A. bicarbonate wasting
B. glycosuria
C. renal failure
D. nephritic syndrome
E. inappropriate antidiuresis
REF. 1, p. 572

736. Which one of the following features is LEAST common in renal amyloidosis?
A. Massive proteinuria not necessarily related to glomerular involvement as estimated from light microscopy
B. Proteinuria which is moderately or poorly selective
C. Severe hypertension
D. Renal vein thrombosis
E. Bence-Jones proteinuria
REF. 10, p. 1529

737. Which of the following clinical manifestations of periarteritis nodosa is LEAST commonly encountered?
A. Predominance in the male
B. Hypertension
C. Proteinuria
D. Polyarthralgia
E. Nephrotic syndrome
REF. 10, p. 1519

738. In considering renal involvement in periarteritis nodosa which of the following factors is NOT correct?
A. Renal involvement is seen in 80 to 90% of the patients
B. The typical presentation of renal involvement is hematuria
C. Telescoped urinary sediment is not seen
D. Disruption of the elastic lamina of the small renal vessels distinguishes the vascular lesions from the lesions secondary to hypertension, where reduplication is seen
E. Progressive renal failure is usually a late manifestation
REF. 10, p. 1519

739. In a patient who had fever, polyarthralgia mononeuritis multiplex, and testicular pain, which of the following is NOT correct?
A. The typical renal presentation is hematuria
B. Nephrotic syndrome is unusual
C. Hypertension is unusual
D. Renal failure usually occurs late
E. Amphetamine abuse and hepatitis may cause this illness
REF. 10, p. 1519

740. A 40-year-old man develops myalgias, fever, edema, and severe oliguria, followed by paralysis of the left radial and right median nerves. Renal biopsy shows which one of the following?
A. Total glomerular sclerosis
B. Diffuse mesangial proliferation
C. Diffuse and focal glomerulosclerosis
D. Crescents and focal fibrinoid necrosis and proliferation
E. Glomerular birefringence under ultraviolet light
REF. 1, p. 535

741. The most common finding in the glomerulus of polyarteritis nodosa is
A. fibrinoid necrosis
B. immune deposit deposition
C. reduplication of the elastic lamina
D. crescent formation
E. interstitial inflammation
REF. 10, p. 1519

742. A young woman presenting with severe uremia and oliguria had noted abdominal pain, hematuria, and arthritis 4 weeks earlier. Two days after the first hemodialysis a fine purpuric rash appeared on the buttocks, knees, and elbows. In this patient, whose renal function recovered partially after 6 weeks of dialysis, which of the following is NOT correct?
A. The renal biopsy showed diffuse and focal mesangial proliferation, with about 50% crescent formation
B. Electron-dense deposits were seen predominantly in the mesangium
C. Immunofluorescence showed diffuse IgG and complement deposits in a largely peripheral distribution
D. The biopsy of uninvolved skin revealed deposits in the walls of superficial capillaries
E. The value of giving steroids or cytotoxic drugs remains unproven
REF. 10, p. 1511

743. Which one of the following features is LEAST characteristic of renal involvement in anaphylactoid purpura (Henoch-Schönlein syndrome)?
A. Gross hematuria
B. Nephrotic syndrome
C. Reduced serum complement levels
D. Elevated serum IgA levels
E. Recurrent acute nephritis syndrome, apparently related to food allergy
REF. 10, p. 1511

744. The renal findings in anaphylactoid purpura suggest which one of the following as the most likely pathogenetic mechanism?
A. A diffuse vasculitis with renal involvement
B. An immune-complex disease involving activation of classic complement pathway
C. A reaction to the development of antibasement membrane antibodies
D. Direct viral involvement with possibly secondary immunologic reactions
E. An immune-complex disease with activation of the alternate complement pathway
REF. 10, p. 1512

745. A young woman with nephrotic syndrome has normal complement, antinuclear antibody and antistreptolysin titers, but renal biopsy shows extramembranous glomerulopathy and mesangial deposits. The most likely diagnosis is
A. renal vein thrombosis
B. amyloidosis
C. systemic lupus erythematosus
D. poststreptococcal nephritis
E. carcinoma elsewhere
REF. 10, p. 1503

746. In the immunofluorescent study of the renal lesions in anaphylactoid purpura, which of the following is most characteristic?
A. Diffuse staining with granular deposits of IgA, C3, and properdin
B. Diffuse staining with IgG and C1q
C. Focal deposits of IgA and C1q
D. Segmented paramesangial capillary deposits of IgA and IgG
E. Minimal immunofluorescent staining
REF. 10, p. 1512

747. In considering the renal lesions found in Wegener's granulomatosis, which of the following statements is NOT correct?
A. Of the patients, 80% will have some evidence of renal involvement
B. The renal lesions include diffuse or segmental necrotizing glomerulonephritis accompanied by a granulomatous reaction around blood vessel walls
C. Scattered immunoglobulin and C3 granular deposits may be seen on immunofluorescence
D. Electron-dense deposits may be seen by electron microscopy
E. The poor prognosis is unaffected by present therapy
REF. 10, p. 1522

748. Crescentic glomerulonephritis with renal failure may occur in all EXCEPT which one of the following?
A. Wegener's granulomatosis
B. Exposure to hydrocarbons
C. Henoch-Schönlein purpura
D. Exposure to silica
E. Cimetidine administration
REF. 11(6), pp. 16, 28

749. Which one of the following statements about sickle cell disease is INCORRECT?
A. Small multiple renal infarcts may lead to loss of function of one kidney
B. Papillary necrosis is the usual cause of progression to renal failure
C. A renal tubular defect may cause hyperkalemia and hyperphosphatemia
D. Most patients cannot concentrate their urine to more than 800 mOsm
E. A membranoproliferative glomerulonephritis with splitting of the glomerular basement membrane but normal complement levels may occur
REF. 10, pp. 1703-1705

750. Hematuria in patients with sickle(s) hemoglobin
A. occurs with sickle cell trait but not with the homozygous disease
B. usually comes from the right kidney and subsides spontaneously
C. filling defects are frequently seen on intravenous pyelography and usually represent blood-clots
D. urinary acidification is the treatment of choice
E. early nephrectomy will prevent recurrences and should be employed to reduce transfusion requirements
REF. 7, p. 1236

751. In rheumatoid arthritis a nephrotic syndrome with normal appearing glomeruli on light microscopy is most compatible with
A. gold therapy
B. amyloidosis
C. ibuprofen
D. phenacetin
E. penicillamine
REF. 12(10), p. 170

752. Following gold therapy for rheumatoid arthritis which of the following is LEAST likely?
A. Gold deposition in tubular mitochondria
B. Epimembranous electron-dense deposits
C. Microscopic hematuria
D. Renal failure
E. Toxic dermatitis
REF. 10, p. 2080

753. A 40-year-old male suffering from multiple myeloma for 6 months had been treated intensively with chemotherapy and was admitted to the hospital in a drowsy state. His BUN was 150 mg; creatinine 10 mg; uric acid 12 mg; Na 132 mEq; K 5 mEq; Cl 107; CO_2 16 mmol/L; urine output 300 cc/24 hr. After proper hydration and alkali therapy urine output increased to 400 cc/24 hr. IV mannitol 50 g was given without appreciable effect. Which of the following should be done immediately?

A. IV furosemide 500 mg
B. Allopurinol 100 mg QID po
C. IV acetazolamide 250 mg
D. Dialysis
E. Mannitol 100 g IV

REF. 7, p. 1246

754. Which of the following statements does NOT apply to cirrhotic glomerular sclerosis?

A. It progresses inexorably to produce renal insufficiency
B. It is characterized by an accumulation of PAS-positive fibrillar material in the mesangium and mild proliferation of endothelial cells
C. Immunofluorescence is generally negative, although mesangial IgA, IgG, and C3 deposits have been described
D. Laminated mesangial bodies in the mesangium, and subendothelial particles are seen by electron microscopy
E. Proteinuria is the main clinical manifestation

REF. 10, p. 1534

755. Which one of the following statements regarding multiple myeloma is FALSE?

A. The use of intravenous contrast media must be approached with great caution
B. Defects in urine concentration, acidification, and Fanconi's syndrome may occur
C. Renal amyloidosis is seen most often in light chain myeloma, should be suspected when there is heavy proteinuria, and may respond to colchicine
D. Hypercalcemia, hyperuricemia, interstitial nephropathy, and toxicity from light chains may contribute to renal insufficiency
E. Renal failure is a common cause of death, second only to infection

REF. 1, pp. 571-572

756. Which of the following is LEAST common in the syndrome of homogenous increase in monoclonal IgM associated with lymphoid cell proliferation (Waldenstrom's macroglobulinemia)?
A. Proteinuria
B. Nephrotic syndrome and azotemia
C. Renal amyloidosis
D. Acute renal failure
E. Low molecular weight (Bence Jones) proteinuria
REF. 10, p. 1526

757. Renal disease in myeloma may result from all of the following EXCEPT
A. alpha globulin
B. myeloma protein
C. amyloidosis
D. hypercalciuria
E. Bence Jones protein
REF. 7, p. 1242

758. The renal concentrating defect in multiple myeloma may be the result of
A. Bence Jones protein in the tubular cells
B. hypocalcemia
C. hyperuricemia
D. lack of ADH
E. nephrotic syndrome
REF. 7, p. 1244

759. The most characteristic change of thrombotic thrombocytopenic purpura is
A. endothelial proliferation
B. basement membrane disruption with the production of gaps
C. epithelial crescents
D. eosinophilic hyaline thrombi
E. glomerular necrosis and karyorrhexis
REF. 7, p. 293

760. With respect to renal involvement in thrombotic thrombocytopenic purpura, which of the following statements is FALSE?
A. Renal involvement is frequent but usually mild
B. Complement and fibrinogen levels may be reduced but plasma renin levels may be strikingly elevated
C. Acute renal failure is uncommon but tends to be severe and irreversible
D. Hypertension is unusual and usually transient
E. Recurrence after renal transplantation may occur
REF. 8, p. 568

761. Which one of the following is LEAST likely to be elevated in a 60-year-old woman who has bone pain, anemia, proteinuria, and an abnormal peak on serum protein electrophoresis?
A. Serum uric acid
B. Urinary light chains
C. Serum calcium
D. Serum alkaline phosphatase
E. Blood urea nitrogen
REF. 1, p. 966

762. Which of the following is NOT likely to be associated with homogenous tubular casts surrounded by multinuclear giant cells and nuclear debris?
A. Progressive renal insufficiency
B. Nephrocalcinosis and hyperuricemia
C. Hypertension and hematuria
D. AL fibril amyloidosis
E. Contrast-induced acute renal failure
REF. 10, p. 1656

763. Immune aggregate deposition within the mesangium is compatible with the pathogenesis of the glomerulonephritis associated with which one of the following?
A. Malaria
B. Echinococcus granulosus
C. Immunoglobulin A
D. Hepatitis "e" antigen
E. Thyroglobulin
REF. 11(6), pp. 10-11

764. Which one of the following is LEAST likely to give rise to a nephrotic syndrome characterized histologically by increased cellularity and expansion of mesangial matrix, with a "double-contoured" or "tram-track" appearance of the capillary walls?
A. Carcinoma of the stomach
B. Sickle cell disease
C. Systemic lupus erythematosis
D. Mixed essential cryoglobulinemia
E. Waldenstrom's macroglobulinemia
REF. 10, pp. 1437, 1443

765. Minimal change nephrotic syndrome has been associated with all but which one of the following?
A. Sarcoidosis
B. Thymoma
C. Lithium
D. Hodgkin's disease
E. Ibuprofen
REF. 10, pp. 1420, 1523

766. Which one of the following findings is most likely in a diabetic heroin addict presenting with fever, weight loss, hematuria, proteinuria (1 g/24 hr), and hypocomplementemia?
A. Focal sclerosis and hyalinosis
B. Intercapillary glomerulosclerosis
C. Focal proliferation and necrosis
D. Amyloid deposits
E. Fusion of foot processes only
REF. 10, p. 1536

767. In the hepatorenal syndrome which of the following statements is INCORRECT?
A. Proteinuria is absent or minimal
B. Examination of the urinary sediment may reveal a variety of formed elements
C. Examination of the urinary sediment may reveal few abnormalities
D. Tubule cell casts, often bile-stained, may be seen in the urinary sediment
E. Concentrating ability is lost early
REF. 10, p. 122

768. Renal failure in Laennec cirrhosis is the result of
   A. bile nephrosis
   B. toxic metabolites
   C. circulatory disturbances involving the kidney
   D. tubular necrosis
   E. immune complex deposition
   REF. 7, p. 1306

769. A nephrotic syndrome with carpal tunnel syndrome, neuropathy, cardiac disease, and Fanconi's syndrome is most characteristic of
   A. polyarteritis nodosa
   B. Fabry's disease
   C. amyloidosis
   D. macroglobulinemia
   E. Sjögren's disease
   REF. 10, p. 1528

9. RENAL FAILURE

DIRECTIONS: Each of the questions or incomplete statements below is followed by a list of suggested answers or completions. Select the one that is best in each case.

A. Acute Renal Failure

770. In renal failure from nontraumatic rhabdomyolysis
    A. myoglobin levels are high in the blood
    B. painful muscular swelling is often present but dehydration is unusual
    C. hypercalcemia may occur, but phosphate and urate levels tend to be low
    D. creatinine phosphokinase levels are high, but aldolase and SGPT levels are normal
    E. plasma creatinine may increase by more than 2.5 mg 100 ml/day
    REF. 7, pp. 196

771. A patient with long-standing congestive failure develops acute renal failure following an operation for obstructive jaundice. Hemodialysis becomes necessary, but during the third hour of treatment she is noted to develop ventricular ectonic beats and atrioventricular dissociation. The most likely cause is
    A. dialysis disequilibrium
    B. digitalis intoxication
    C. hard water syndrome
    D. hyperkalemia
    E. myocardial infarction
    REF. 7, p. 435

772. Renal cortical necrosis has all of the following characteristics EXCEPT
A. total anuria is common in the first few days
B. calcification of the renal parenchyma may occur
C. recovery of renal function is uncommon
D. both kidneys are equally involved
E. thrombosis of the large renal arteries is common
REF. 7, p. 194

773. Renal cortical necrosis has been prevented in experimental animals by all of the following measures EXCEPT
A. deep anesthesia
B. denervation of the kidneys
C. ganglion-blocking agents
D. nitrogen mustard before injection of bacterial toxins
E. corticosteroids
REF. 7, p. 199

774. The most common cause of cortical necrosis is
A. severe dehydration
B. septicemia
C. abruptio placentae
D. crush injury
E. burns
REF. 7, p. 144

775. Renal cortical necrosis has all of the following characteristics EXCEPT
A. total anuria is common in the first few days
B. calcification of renal parenchyma may occur
C. recovery of renal function is uncommon
D. both kidneys are equally involved
E. thrombosis of the large renal arteries is common
REF. 7, p. 199

776. The peak loss of fluid from the body following a burn occurs
A. within the first 12 hours
B. on the second day
C. 48 to 72 hours later
D. 5 to 10 days later
E. 14 to 21 days later
REF. 5, (2nd Ed.), p. 1045

777. Silver nitrate therapy of burns may result in
A. hyponatremia
B. hyperkalemia
C. respiratory alkalosis
D. hyperchloremia
E. none of the above
REF. 5 (2nd Ed.), p. 1057

778. Mafemide (Salfamylon) therapy for burns can result in
A. hyperkalemia
B. metabolic acidosis
C. hypernatremia
D. water intoxication
E. inappropriate ADH secretion
REF. 5 (2nd Ed.), p. 1055

779. The electrolyte solution used in burns should be
A. 5% dextrose/water
B. 2.5% dextrose/half strength normal saline
C. normal saline
D. lactate Ringer's solution
E. Ringer's solution
REF. 5, (2nd Ed.), p. 1052

780. Acute renal failure with rhabdomyolysis may be associated with all of the following EXCEPT
A. pentazocine and tripelennamine injection
B. carbon monoxide poisoning
C. vascular occlusion
D. alcoholism
E. gentamicin
REF. 11(1), p. 260

781. Acute renal failure and hepatotoxicity are classically seen with
A. bichloride of mercury
B. methyl alcohol
C. carbon tetrachloride
D. lead
E. cadmium
REF. 7, p. 1450

782. The most frequent cause of death in acute renal failure is
A. uremia
B. pulmonary edema
C. hyperkalemia
D. infection
E. hyponatremia
REF. 2, p. 1610

783. Which of the following is most consistent with acute tubular necrosis?
A. U/P urea > 20:1
B. U/P creatinine = 5:1
C. U/P osmol > 2:1
D. U Na = 12 mEq/L
E. Urinary specific gravity = 1.025
REF. 2, p. 1608

784. Which of the following is LEAST likely to cause renal failure?
A. Vancomycin
B. Methicillin
C. Cephalosporins
D. Streptomycin
E. Gentamicin
REF. 7, pp. 1453-1454

785. Acute renal failure associated with which of the following agents may also cause severe gastritis and GI bleeding?
A. Phosphorus
B. Chloroform
C. Potassium chloride
D. Mercuric chloride
E. Chromium
REF. 7, p. 1446

786. Concerning acute renal failure from bichloride of mercury ingestion, which of the following is FALSE?
A. Hemodialysis and dimercaprol are the preferred methods of treatment
B. Ulceration of the palate is frequently observed
C. Oxalate crystals are frequently found in the renal tubules
D. Circulatory failure is frequently observed, and jaundice occurs in one-third of the patients
E. Rectal bleeding is a serious delayed complication and may require emergency colectomy
REF. 7, p. 1446

787. Match the following:
A. Lead
B. Organic mercurials
C. Cadmium
D. Ethylene glycol
E. Amphotericin

1. Calcium oxalate crystals
2. Nephrotic syndrome
3. Hypertension
4. Aminoaciduria
5. Renal tubular acidosis
REF. 3, p. 1100

788. Which of the following is NOT a characteristic finding of ethylene glycol ingestion and ARF within 48 hours?
A. Flank pain
B. Proteinuria
C. Oxalate crystaluria
D. Metabolic acidosis
E. Ethylene glycol in the urine
REF. 7, p. 1450

789. Which of the following is NOT related to the development of obstructive uropathy?
A. Cyclophosphamide
B. Indomethacin
C. Sulfonamides
D. Warfarin
E. Methysergide
REF. 7, p. 877

790. Which of the following parts of nephron is most likely to be damaged in nephrotoxic-induced acute renal failure?
A. Glomerulus
B. Proximal tubule
C. Distal tubule
D. Collecting tubule
E. Loop of Henle
REF. 7, p. 176

791. Acute worsening of azotemia in patients with acute renal failure receiving tetracycline therapy (other than doxycycline) may be due to
A. direct nephrotoxic effect
B. decreased renal blood flow
C. prevention of amino acid utilization for protein synthesis
D. increased protein breakdown
E. tubular obstruction
REF. 12(6), p. 131

792. Which of the following is true in acute tubular necrosis?
A. Most patients excrete less than 10 ml of urine/24 hr
B. Urinary sodium concentration commonly exceeds 40 mEq/L
C. Urine osmolality exceeds plasma osmolality severalfold
D. Urine output usually increases markedly following fluid replacement and mannitol infusion
E. Some of the lowest urine volumes occur in patients with burns
REF. 8, p. 394

793. In acute renal failure, anuria is LEAST consistent with
A. acute cortical necrosis
B. rapidly progressive glomerulonephritis
C. gentamicin-induced renal failure
D. postirradiation uremia in chronic myeloid leukemia
E. bilateral renal artery emboli
REF. 7, p. 169

794. Which of the following measures reduces the nephrotoxicity of amphoterecin-B?
A. Alkalinization of urine
B. Intravenous mannitol
C. Steroids
D. Intravenous potassium chloride
E. None of the above
REF. 12(6), p. 132

795. Regarding fluid balance in acute renal failure
A. an indwelling urethral catheter is essential to accurately manage fluid balance
B. fluid balance is best maintained by an indwelling catheter in the inferior vena cava
C. patients should be weighed daily and allowed to gain 1 kg/day
D. sodium is best administered as hypertonic saline, to avoid hyponatremia and fluid overload
E. the basal requirement for a 70 kg man is about 400 ml/24 hr
REF. 7, p. 184

796. A patient with multiple myeloma who had been treated with melphalan is transferred for treatment of acute renal failure. His BUN is 200 mg%, potassium level 8 mEq/L. Which of the following measures should be instituted first?
A. Immediate treatment with allopurinol
B. Immediate retrograde pyelogram
C. Pelvic lavage with sodium bicarbonate
D. Administration of glucose, insulin, and sodium bicarbonate
E. Hemodialysis
REF. 7, p. 185

797. All of the following changes take place during severe prerenal azotemia EXCEPT
A. glomerular filtration and renal blood flow decrease
B. reabsorption of sodium by the proximal tubules decreases
C. renal blood flow is redistributed from the cortex to the corticomedullary region
D. the concentration of urea in the urine increases
E. the epithelium of the cortical collecting duct becomes more permeable to water
REF. 7, p. 177

798. Which of the following changes take place during acute arterial hypotension?
A. Cortical renal blood flow increases from 50% to 90% of the total renal blood flow
B. Cortical renal blood flow decreases by 30% of its initial value
C. Cortical renal blood flow decreases from 80% to about 10% of the total renal blood flow
D. Corticomedullary blood flow increases from 10% to 20% of the total renal blood flow
E. Corticomedullary blood flow remains unchanged
REF. 7, p. 181

799. Which of the following is LEAST likely to cause renal failure?
A. Chloramphenicol
B. Methicillin
C. Rifampin
D. Kanamycin
E. Gentamicin
REF. 7, p. 1453

800. Early renal vasoconstriction in myohemoglobinuric acute renal failure can be reversed by which of the following measures?
A. Intravenous fluid administration
B. Diuretics
C. Alkalinization of blood
D. Dialysis
E. Vasodilator drug therapy
REF. 12(6), p. 251

801. Which of the following tests will be most helpful in establishing a diagnosis of ethylene glycol ingestion producing renal failure?
A. Urine for ethylene glycol
B. Ethylene glycol blood level
C. Urine for oxalic acid
D. Urine sediment shows hexagonal crystals
E. Renal biopsy
REF. 1, p. 561

802. Which of the following measures has been relatively most effective in the treatment of acute renal failure from hepatorenal syndrome?
A. Dopamine infusion
B. Prostaglandin infusion
C. Exchange transfusion
D. Dialysis
E. LeVeen peritoneovenous shunt
REF. 12(6), p. 260

803. In which type of acute renal failure is the toxic agent potentiated by alcohol?
A. Methyl alcohol
B. Arsenic
C. Carbon tetrachloride
D. Ethylene glycol
E. Propylene glycol
REF. 7, p. 1450

804. In which kind of acute renal failure is severe gastrointestinal hemorrhage seen most frequently?
A. Phosphorus
B. Chloroform
C. Potassium chlorate
D. Mercuric chloride
E. Chromium
REF. 7, p. 1444

805. Renal medullary necrosis is most frequently seen
A. following the liberation of pancreatic enzymes into the blood stream
B. in the hepatorenal syndrome
C. in elderly diabetic patients
D. in patients with sickle cell disease
E. in patients with interstitial lead nephritis
REF. 7, p. 1211

806. Which of the following laboratory parameters is most helpful in diagnosing acute tubular necrosis?
A. Urinary sodium concentration
B. Serum blood urea nitrogen and creatinine ratio
C. Urine osmolality
D. Fractional excretion of filtered sodium
E. Renal failure index
REF. 8, p. 396

807. During the diuretic phase of an acute renal failure vasopressin is administered to reduce the urine flow. The effect of vasopressin under such circumstances will
A. decrease urine flow without change in urine osmolality
B. increase urine osmolality by 30% but no change in urine flow
C. decrease urine osmolality
D. have no effect on urine flow and osmolality
E. increase urine flow and osmolality
REF. 7, p. 173

808. A patient, weighing 60 kg, with acute renal failure is in oliguric stage, passing 450 cc of urine/24 hr, has a temp of 100.6°F, normal fluid volume, normal BP and pulmonary capillary wedge pressure. The 24 hr fluid requirement is approximately how many cc?
A. 500
B. 700
C. 1000
D. 1200
E. 1800
REF. 7, p. 184

809. Which of the following is probably the most important factor in the pathogenesis of the delayed wound healing frequently observed in acute renal failure?
A. Electrolyte imbalance
B. Associated infection and toxemia
C. Anemia and decreased erythropoiesis
D. Inhibition of fibroblast proliferation
E. Depleted vitamin C stores
REF. 10, p. 1189

810. Complete anuria for more than 48 hours may suggest
A. acute tubular necrosis
B. bilateral renal arterial embolism
C. severe prerenal azotemia
D. acute or chronic renal failure
E. drug-induced interstitial nephritis
REF. 2, p. 1608

811. Low urine Na (below 10 mEq/L) is found in
A. acute tubular necrosis
B. cortical necrosis
C. Addison's disease
D. chronic glomerulonephritis
E. terminal hepatic failure
REF. 2, p. 1612

812. A patient with long-standing congestive heart failure develops acute renal failure following an operation for obstructive jaundice. Hemodialysis became necessary but during the third hour of treatment she is noted to develop chills and translucent blood in the venous line. The most likely cause is
A. dialysis disequilibrium
B. hard water syndrome
C. hyperkalemia
D. digitalis intoxication
E. copper intoxication
REF. 10, p. 2334

813. In a typical patient with oliguria in acute renal failure, the rate of excretion of filtered Na is
A. 0.5%
B. 7%
C. 15%
D. 20%
E. 2%
REF. 1, p. 498

814. Acute renal failure in myeloma is most commonly caused by
A. hypercalcemia
B. hyperuricemia
C. tubular blockage by Bence Jones protein
D. plasma cell infiltration
E. hyperviscosity
REF. 1, p. 966

815. In managing a patient with acute renal failure the following laboratory data are obtained: BUN-100%; serum creatinine - 12 mg%; serum sodium 125 mEq/L; serum potassium 6 mEq/L; urine sodium 50 mEq/L; urine creatinine 24 mg%; urine potassium 20 mEq/L. What is the fractional excretion of filtered sodium?
A. 2
B. 5
C. 10
D. 20
E. 25
REF. 7, p. 396

816. In the presence of life-threatening hyperkalemia the most rapidly effective method for treating cardiac toxicity is
A. immediate peritoneal dialysis
B. infusion of sodium bicarbonate
C. intravenous therapy with glucose and bicarbonate
D. infusion with calcium gluconate
E. cationic exchange resins both orally and per rectum
REF. 10, p. 1196

817. The last function to recover after acute renal failure is
A. acidification
B. concentration
C. dilution
D. sodium conservation
E. amino acid reabsorption
REF. 5, p. 772

B. Chronic Renal Failure

818. Which of the following statements are true about the trade-off hypothesis?
A. Middle molecules are preferentially retained to aid excretion of highly toxic, low molecular weight substances
B. Secondary hyperparathyroidism averts the development of osteomalacia
C. Parathormone hypersecretion causes the retention of phosphate
D. Secretion of natriuretic substance may avoid sodium retention
E. Some nephrons are preferentially shut down to maintain the function of others
REF. 8, p. 432

819. The smallest amount of urine that can normally clear the blood of its metabolites is
A. 100 cc
B. 500 cc
C. 1000 cc
D. 1500 cc
E. 50 cc
REF. 3, p. 1072

820. Which of the following statements is FALSE?
A. The digoxin dose in most uremic patients is 0.125 mg on alternate days
B. The dose of procainamide in uremia is unchanged
C. For propranolol little dose modification is required in uremia
D. Lidocaine in uremia is given in normal doses
E. The dose of quinidine in uremia is unchanged
REF 7, p. 523

821. In the anephric patient aldosterone secretion is predominantly regulated by
A. ACTH
B. sodium balance
C. posture
D. water balance
E. potassium
REF. 7, p. 1619

822. The metabolic clearance rate of aldosterone in patients with end-stage renal disease is
A. normal
B. low
C. high
D. increased with nephrectomy
E. unknown
REF. 10, p. 2176

823. If a patient with advanced renal failure excretes 900 mOsm solute daily, his urine volume will be about
A. 900 cc
B. equal to intake
C. 4500 cc
D. 3000 cc
E. 450 cc
REF. 5, p. 804

824. In the presence of chronic renal failure, which of the following statements is FALSE?
A. Uric acid clearance tends to fall more profoundly than the creatinine clearance
B. Hyperuricemia almost always occurs when the BUN level rises about 100 mg/100 ml
C. Tubular secretion of uric acid is reduced less than tubular reabsorption
D. Clinical "secondary" gout is unusual
E. The blood level of uric acid is particularly high in lead nephropathy
REF. 7, p. 231

825. Diminution in urine volume in chronic renal failure usually signifies
A. increased ADH release
B. diminished diluting ability
C. increased solute load
D. diminished GFR
E. tubular damage greater than glomerular damage
REF. 5, p. 811

826. Which of the following is most likely to accelerate the progression of renal failure in a patient with chronic glomerulonephritis?
A. Hypertension
B. Hematuria
C. Hyperuricemia
D. A salt-losing state
E. Sensitivity to furosemide
REF. 2, p. 1642

827. Which of the following is most consistent with a history of excessive milk of magnesia ingestion in a chronic dialysis patient?
A. Dysphasia, myoclonus, delirium
B. Nystagmus, ataxia, confusion
C. Confusion, excitement, hyperreflexia
D. Muscle weakness, hyporeflexia, quadriplegia
E. Tremor, hyporeflexia, scanning speech
REF. 7, p. 1651

828. In the dialysis disequilibrium syndrome
A. water moves out of the cells
B. changes are more marked with slow dialysis
C. hypermagnesemia is a factor
D. brain pH may fall
E. brain water is unchanged
REF. 7, p. 443

829. The use of acetate in the dialysis bath may result in all of the following EXCEPT
A. difficulties when small dialyzers are used
B. acidosis from bicarbonate removal
C. myocardial depression
D. conversion to fatty acids and triglycerides
E. conversion to cholesterol
REF. 5, p. 853

830. Which of the following is NOT a complication of uremia?
A. Hemiparesis
B. Papilledema
C. Coma
D. Asterixis
E. Myoclonus
REF. 10, p. 2306

831. Which is NOT a sign of dialysis disequilibrium?
A. Hemiparesis
B. Headache
C. Convulsions
D. Muscle cramps
E. Nausea
REF. 10, p. 2507

832. Inability to conserve sodium in chronic renal failure is due to
A. obligatory wastage of sodium to maintain the acid-base balance
B. defective reabsorption of sodium because of tubular damage
C. an osmotic diuresis in each functioning nephron
D. an obligatory increase in blood volume depressing reabsorption
E. inhibition of aldosterone production
REF. 13, p. 497

833. In chronic renal failure
A. excretion of ammonium ions is normal
B. excretion of titratable acid and ammonium is increased
C. ammonium excretion is more impaired than titratable acid excretion
D. excretion of ammonium and titratable acidity excretion are normal
E. titratable acid excretion is more impaired than ammonium excretion
REF. 7, p. 501

834. Which of the following is NOT a complication of uremia?
A. Anemia
B. Pericarditis
C. Peripheral neuropathy
D. Pruritis
E. Hepatitis
REF. 10, p. 2503

835. In chronic renal failure, free water clearance, when expressed per 100 ml GFR
A. is frequently within normal range
B. is high
C. is low
D. increases with progressive destruction of nephrons
E. none of the above
REF. 7, p. 497

836. Factors responsible for growth failure in uremic children include all of the following EXCEPT
A. acidosis
B. anemia
C. polyuria
D. osteodystrophy
E. neuropathy
REF. 13, p. 856

837. Which of the following findings is most suggestive of pericardial tamponade in a maintenance dialysis patient?
A. Increased pulse rate on deep inspiration
B. The sudden accumulation of ascites
C. The disappearance of a previously heard pericardial rub
D. Hypotension during dialysis ultrafiltration
E. A poorly palpable cardiac impulse
REF. 7, p. 271

838. Which of the following does NOT exaggerate the electrocardiographic abnormalities of hyperkalemia?
A. Hypernatremia
B. Hypocalcemia
C. Acidosis
D. Hypermagnesemia
E. Hyponatremia
REF. 5, p. 153

839. Which of the following statements is true of uremic pericarditis?
A. In untreated uremics it is uncommon if the BUN level is below 80 mg/100 ml
B. Pain in the chest is generally absent
C. Effusions rarely exist for many weeks in patients on dialysis
D. Bloody effusions are rare
E. Most patients eventually develop tamponade
REF. 2, p. 1617

840. Which is NOT an accepted treatment for pericarditis?
A. Prolonging dialysis
B. Anticoagulants
C. Pericardial window
D. Pericardial stripping
E. Pericardial aspiration
REF. 2, p. 1617

841. Which of the following correlates best with pericarditis occurring several months after starting hemodialysis therapy?
A. Plasma urea level
B. Patients who are dialyzed infrequently
C. Creatinine clearance
D. Guanidine level in blood
E. Duration of chronic renal failure
REF. 1, p. 504

842. Which of the following findings is LEAST suggestive of pericardial effusion in a maintenance hemodialysis patient?
A. Decreased pulse rate
B. Sudden accumulation of ascites
C. Disappearance of previously heard pericardial rub
D. Severe hypotension during dialysis ultrafiltration
E. A poorly palpable carotid pulse
REF. 7, p. 270

843. In maintenance dialysis of patients with peripheral neuropathy the most important etiological factor appears to be
A. the height of the blood urea level
B. the residual urinary output
C. the duration of uremia before dialysis is begun
D. protein malnutrition and vitamin deficiency
E. accumulation of methylguanidine and guanidinosuccinic acid
REF. 7, p. 380

844. Which of the following features is LEAST compatible with the peripheral neuropathy of chronic renal failure?
A. Footdrop
B. Sensory loss in the lower extremities
C. Wristdrop
D. Restless leg syndrome
E. Burning feet syndrome
REF. 7, p. 379

845. Although symptomatic neuropathy used to be seen frequently in patients with chronic renal failure, symptomatic neuropathy is now seen only rarely at the start of dialysis therapy. Possible reasons for this change include all EXCEPT
A. early onset of dialysis
B. increased frequency of dialysis
C. improved dialysis availability
D. change in dialyzing membrane
E. change in vitamin replacement therapy
REF. 7, p. 380

846. Which of the following drugs causes neuropathy in uremic patients?
A. Vibramycin
B. Chloromycetin
C. Trimethoprim
D. Nitrofurantoin
E. Cephalosporins
REF. 7, p. 380

847. Which of the following is true for uremic neuropathy?
A. Asymptomatic neuropathy occurs in about 50% of patients with end-stage renal failure or on dialysis
B. Vitamin B_1 reverses the symptoms
C. Nerve conduction velocity is within normal limits
D. Special tests for cutaneous sensations are normal
E. Only motor conduction velocity test is required to make the diagnosis
REF. 7, p. 377

848. Which of the following statements does NOT apply to uremic neuropathy?
A. In the early stages, sensory changes are more marked than motor changes
B. Nerve conduction times may be depressed even when clinical neuropathy is absent
C. Motor paralysis is often helped by renal transplantation but rarely by dialysis
D. The earliest manifestations occur in the upper extremities
E. An asymmetrical neuritis has been described following rapid ultrafiltration
REF. 7, p. 351

849. The most effective therapy for severe uremic peripheral neuropathy is
A. phenytoin
B. increasing dialysis time
C. thiamine
D. renal transplantation
E. sodium bicarbonate
REF. 7, p. 381

850. Which of the following is FALSE in the case of a dialysis patient with radiologic changes of osteodystrophy who has a serum calcium level of 10 mg/100 ml and a phosphate level of 7.2 mg/100 ml?
A. Despite claims to the contrary she is not taking her aluminum hydroxide gel
B. She should undergo parathyroidectomy
C. Vitamin D administration may be hazardous in this patient
D. Oral calcium supplements alone will not help her bone disease
E. Increasing the calcium concentration in the dialysate to 9 mg/100 ml will suppress parathyroid activity and help heal her bone disease
REF. 7, p. 351

851. Regarding renal osteodystrophy, which of the following statements is FALSE?
A. Intestinal absorption of calcium is usually impaired
B. Parathormone levels are invariably high
C. The optimal dialysate calcium level is 5 mg%
D. Treatment with aluminum hydroxide will reduce hyperphosphatemia
E. High magnesium levels suppress parathyroid activity
REF. 7, p. 435

852. The most important cause of metastatic calcification in chronic renal failure is
A. hypercalcemia
B. acidosis
C. hyperphosphatemia
D. hypervitaminosis D
E. none of the above
REF. 7, p. 343

853. Which one of the following is LEAST likely to improve bone disease seen in a chronic dialysis patient?
A. Low phosphate diet
B. Parathyroidectomy
C. 25- OH vitamin D_3
D. Aluminum hydroxide
E. 1,25 OH vitamin D_3
REF. 7, pp. 361-362

854. Rugger Jersey spine in chronic renal failure is due to
A. osteomalacia
B. osteoporosis
C. osteitis fibrosa
D. osteosclerosis
E. none of the above
REF. 7, p. 328

855. Regarding the thyroid status of maintenance dialysis patients
A. TSH levels are invariably high, indicating retention by the kidney rather than hypothyroidism
B. T_4 levels are usually low and T_3 normal
C. a low T_3 is probably an indication for thyroid replacement
D. low T_4 and elevated TSH level may be an indication for thyroid replacement
E. conversion of T_4 to T_3 is normal
REF. 7, p. 244

856. Which of the following is true regarding growth hormone in patients with chronic renal failure?
A. Plasma growth hormone is below normal in CRF
B. Growth hormone has no effect on renal function
C. Administration of glucose increases the growth hormone level
D. Glucagon administration decreases growth hormone level
E. All of the above are true
REF. 10, p. 2171

857. All of the following are true regarding gastrin level in chronic renal failure EXCEPT
A. gastrin level is high
B. gastrin level increases
C. there is correlation between basal acid secretions and gastrin level
D. hypercalcemia stimulates gastrin secretion
E. kidney helps in degradation of gastrin
REF. 10, p. 2175

858. Which of the following gastrointestinal abnormalities associated with CRF is NOT improved with dialysis treatment?
A. Uremic gastritis
B. Uremic fetor
C. Peptic ulcer disease
D. Uremic colitis
E. Nausea and vomiting
REF. 3, p. 1618

859. In chronic renal failure salt excretion may increase
A. when there is volume depletion
B. when there is hyponatremia
C. as GFR is progressively decreased
D. when there is nausea and vomiting
E. none of the above
REF. 10, p. 1603

860. Dialysis dementia syndrome includes all of the following clinical features EXCEPT
A. dysparaxia
B. myoclonus
C. seizure
D. reversal of symptoms with vitamin B_{12} therapy
E. normal pressure hydrocepheus
REF. 2, p. 1618

861. The mortality of chronic dialysis is approximately 10%/yr with cardiovascular complications the major cause. Which of the following is also a frequent cause of death in such patients?
A. Sepsis
B. Neuropathy
C. Cerebrovascular disease
D. Metabolic disorders
E. Anemia
REF. 2, p. 261

862. The most common abnormality in dialysis patients is elevation of
A. cholesterol
B. fatty acids
C. phospholipids
D. high-density lipoproteins
E. trilycerides
REF. 7, p. 238

863. In maintenance dialysis patients'
A. testosterone levels are low
B. luteinizing levels are normal but prolactin levels are low
C. TSH levels are increased and T3 levels are normal
D. spermatogenesis is normal
E. TSH levels are reduced
REF. 7, p. 246

864. Plasma parathyroid hormone levels in chronic renal failure correlate well with
A. blood urea nitrogen
B. serum calcium concentration
C. serum magnesium concentration
D. 1,25-dihydroxycholecalciferol levels
E. calcium phosphate product
REF. 13, p. 503

865. Which of the following is NOT improved or corrected by dialysis?
A. Pericarditis
B. Anemia
C. Hypertension
D. Dialysis dementia
E. Prolonged bleeding time
REF. 7, p. 386

866. The half-life of insulin in renal failure is prolonged because
A. the kidney is the main site of insulin degradation
B. excretion of insulin is impaired
C. of peripheral antagonism of insulin action
D. uremia impairs peripheral degradation of insulin
E. degradation in the liver is impaired
REF. 13, p. 505

867. Carbohydrate tolerance in uremia is often impaired. Which of the following statements is FALSE?
A. Basal levels of immunoreactive insulin are elevated
B. Uremic patients are intolerant to both oral and intravenous glucose
C. The response to intravenously administered insulin is blunted
D. The hyperglycemia is due to defective insulin secretion and not to insulin antagonism
E. Basal growth hormone levels are elevated, and the response to glucose is paradoxical
REF. 7, p. 237

868. Regarding the use of antibiotics in end-stage renal failure which of the following may be administered in normal doses?
A. Sulfisoxazole
B. Chloramphenicol
C. Gentamicin
D. Nitrofurantoin
E. Nalidixic acid
REF. 7, p. 523

869. Sodium phenytoin (diphenylhydantoin)
A. is removed by dialysis in significant amounts
B. accumulates in renal failure
C. is bound to protein to a greater extent in uremia
D. has an increased half-life in uremia
E. is potentiated by isoniazid
REF. 7, p. 527

870. Adequacy of bone marrow iron stores in dialysis patients is best evaluated by determining
A. the mean corpuscular hemoglobin concentration
B. ferritin
C. erythropoetin
D. siderophyllin and transferrin
E. serum iron and total iron binding capacity
REF. 7, p. 288

871. Chronic renal failure with significant proteinuria is unlikely to be present in any of the following EXCEPT
A. polycystic kidney
B. obstructive nephropathy
C. malignant nephrosclerosis
D. medullary cystic disease
E. analgesic nephropathy
REF. 2, p. 1597

872. As glomerular filtration rate diminishes, in order to maintain sodium balance
A. fractional sodium excretion decreases
B. fractional sodium excretion must increase
C. fractional sodium excretion must remain constant
D. sodium filtration must increase
E. aldosterone must be inhibited
REF. 1, p. 502

873. The major mechanism of acidosis in chronic renal failure is
A. loss of titratable acids in urine
B. bicarbonaturia
C. reduced tubular ammonia production
D. increased dietary acid intake
E. none of the above
REF. 7, p. 230

874. Rapid correction of systemic acidosis in chronic renal failure by administration of bicarbonate may cause respiratory alkalosis because
A. bicarbonate diffuses slowly into the CSF
B. toxic products continue to accumulate in spite of correction of blood pH
C. osmolality in CSF remains higher than plasma
D. transfer of K^+ into the intracellular space
E. activation of Na^+ - K^+ ATPase enzyme
REF. 1, p. 494

875. In chronic renal failure, most of the acid is buffered by
A. ammonia
B. new bicarbonate synthesis
C. increased titratable acid
D. bone
E. red cells
REF. 7, p. 230

876. Which of the following treatments is most effective in controlling accelerated hypertension of a patient who is on maintenance hemodialysis three times a week and had gained 7 lbs ?
A. Lasix
B. Aprestine
C. Diazoxide
D. Ultrafiltration
E. Beta blockers
REF. 2, p. 1505

877. A patient with chronic renal failure being treated with intravenous penicillin therapy becomes obtunded and has a seizure on the seventh day of treatment. Renal function was unchanged. Next step of treatment should be
A. hemodialysis
B. peritoneal dialysis
C. dilantin
D. discontinue penicillin
E. none of the above
REF. 7, p. 371

878. In a maintenance dialysis patient who develops epilepsy and tuberculosis
A. the dose of ethambutol should be unchanged
B. the dose of phenytoin must be increased because isoniazid accelerates its metabolism
C. the dose of phenytoin must be decreased because it ordinarily is excreted by the kidney
D. the dose of rifampin should be unchanged
E. the dose of isoniazid may need to be increased
REF. 7, p. 525

879. In nonoliguric chronic renal failure, hyperkalemia does not usually occur because
A. there is more secretion of potassium from the proximal renal tubule
B. there is less sodium to be reabsorbed from the tubules since there is a fall of the GFR resulting in less competition fór potassium exchange
C. there is a relatively large amount of hydrogen ion that may be secreted
D. increased flow of high concentration of impermeant anions, sulfate, and phosphate encourages secretion of potassium
E. none of the above
REF. 2, p. 1606

880. Presence of hypokalemia in chronic renal failure is associated with all of the following EXCEPT
   A. poor dietary K+ intake
   B. gastrointestinal loss of K+
   C. excessive diuretic therapy
   D. Fanconi's syndrome
   E. renal tubular acidosis type IV
   REF. 2, p. 1616

881. Respiratory alkalosis may occur in chronic renal failure with acidosis following
   A. fast peritoneal dialysis with no static phase
   B. fast hemodialysis
   C. forced diuresis
   D. IV acetazolamide
   E. IV insulin and glucose
   REF. 1, p. 511

882. Which of the following statements about the hematologic changes in chronic renal failure are FALSE?
   A. Anemia is usually due to lack of bone marrow activity
   B. Burr cells and helmet cells may be due to a microangiopathic hemolytic anemia
   C. A qualitative platelet defect is common
   D. Transfusions should be given to maintain a normal hematocrit
   E. Transfusions are not contraindicated
   REF. 7, p. 287

883. Which of the following statements about bilateral nephrectomy is true?
   A. Transfusion requirements are decreased
   B. Erythropoetin secretion increases
   C. Osteodystrophy often improves
   D. Extrarenal erythropoetin secretion may occur
   E. Hemolysis may increase
   REF. 7, p. 478

884. Erythrocytosis is most likely to be associated with
   A. thrombotic thrombocytopenic purpura
   B. hepatorenal syndrome
   C. transplant rejection
   D. nail-patella syndrome
   E. cystinosis
   REF. 7, p. 285

885. Which of the following hematological complications of chronic renal failure tends to improve after dialysis therapy?
A. Lymphocytopenia
B. Splenomegaly
C. Normocytic normochromic anemia
D. Bleeding diathesis
E. Increased susceptibility to infection
REF. 2, p. 1618

886. Abnormalities of platelet function seen in uremic patients appear to be
A. caused by abnormal platelet production
B. caused by blood urea nitrogen interference with platelet function
C. caused by defective ADP-induced release of platelet factor 3 and defective ADP-induced platelet aggregation
D. abnormalities not corrected by hemodialysis but corrected by peritoneal dialysis
E. abnormalities not corrected by renal transplant
REF. 7, p. 281

887. Which of the following is an indication for blood transfusion for anemia in patients with chronic renal failure when hematocrit is above 25%?
A. Peripheral neuropathy
B. General weakness
C. Macrocytic anemia
D. Angina pectoris
E. Unresponsive to iron therapy
REF. 1, p. 509

888. In chronic renal failure
A. fibrinogen level is usually low
B. fibrinolytic activity is usually increased
C. fibrinolytic activity is restored to normal with regular dialysis
D. fibrinogen remains abnormal even with regular dialysis
E. none of the above
REF. 1, p. 504

889. Solute clearances with peritoneal dialysis may be decreased in all but which of the following?
A. Acute cortical necrosis
B. Scleroderma
C. Diabetes mellitus
D. Heat stroke
E. Malignant hypertension
REF. 7, p. 455

890. The bleeding tendency of uremic patients is most likely due to
A. thrombocytosis
B. marrow dysfunction
C. factor IX deficiency
D. a defect of platelet factor 3
E. thrombocytopenia
REF. 7, p. 280

891. Polyacrylonitrile membranes in dialyzers
A. enhance urea removal
B. are most useful when urea clearance exceeds the blood flow rate
C. decrease water removal by ultrafiltration
D. are not useful for middle-molecule removal
E. increase inulin clearance
REF. 7, p. 453

892. When the concentration of solute in the inflowing dialysate is zero
A. clearance becomes dissociated from dialysance
B. clearance is higher than dialysance
C. clearance is lower than dialysance
D. clearance equals dialysance
E. both clearance and dialysance become zero
REF. 7, p. 450

893. Water in hemodialysis is predominantly removed by
A. solvent drag
B. dialysance
C. diffusion
D. osmotic transfer
E. ultrafiltration
REF. 7, p. 451

894. Which of the following drugs requires a major reduction in dosage in uremia?
A. Gentamicin
B. Lincomycin
C. Nafcillin
D. Oxacillin
E. Novobiocin
REF. 7, p. 523

895. Which of the following drugs is significantly removed during peritoneal dialysis?
A. Kanamycin
B. Vancomycin
C. Tetracycline
D. Chloramphenicol
E. Methicillin
REF. 7, p. 523

896. Which of the following substances has the LOWEST clearance across the peritoneum?
A. Urea
B. Potassium
C. Sodium
D. Creatinine
E. Uric acid
REF. 5, p. 862

897. Hyperosmolarity following peritoneal dialysis is usually a result of
A. too much fluid removal
B. use of hypertonic glucose solutions
C. use of hypertonic sodium solutions
D. use of too little fluid in each exchange
E. use of too rapid changes
REF. 5, p. 865

898. In end-stage renal disease sequential ultrafiltration followed by dialysis
A. makes blood pressure control more difficult
B. improves peripheral neuropathy
C. facilitates middle-molecule removal
D. may produce pericarditis
E. may control ascites
REF. 7, p. 443

899. Which of the following doses is INCORRECT in a patient with a creatinine clearance of 5 ml/min?
A. Ampicillin 500 mg bid
B. Gentamicin 15 mg/8 hr
C. Cephalothin 0. 5 g bid
D. Chloramphenicol 250 mg qid
E. Carbenicillin 5 g/4 hr
REF. 7, p. 552

900. Constipation in chronic dialysis patients is most likely and frequently caused by
A. intramural hematoma from an increased bleeding tendency
B. guanethidine and alpha-methyldopa
C. aluminum hydroxide
D. low-protein diet
E. potassium-binding resins
REF. 7, p. 241

901. Which of the following statements about hemodialysis is FALSE?
A. Fluid is removed mainly by ultrafiltration
B. Solutes are removed mainly by diffusion
C. The removal of larger molecules depends mainly on the surface urea of the dialyzer and the time of dialysis
D. A rapid blood and dialysate flow rate enhances urea removal
E. The permeability of the membrane depends only on the pore size and very little on fluid film or flow path
REF. 7, p. 431

902. Gynecomastia in a maintenance dialysis patient is thought to be due to
A. spironolactone
B. hypothalamic hyperactivity
C. a phenomenon similar to refeeding gynecomastia
D. liver disease
E. parathyroid hyperplasia
REF. 7, p. 246

903. In dialysate regenerating systems, zirconium phosphate reabsorbs which of the following substances?
A. Ammonia
B. Creatinine
C. Uric acid
D. Salicylates
E. Urea
REF. 5, p. 859

904. Which of the following statements about the urea clearance of hemodialyzers is FALSE?
A. Urea clearances increase with the blood flow
B. Urea clearances increase with the dialysate flow
C. For each dialyzer there is a point beyond which the clearance no longer increases, despite increasing blood or dialysate flow
D. Hydrostatic pressure is a minor factor in determining urea clearance
E. Osmosis is a major factor in determining urea clearance
REF. 10, p. 2483

905. Copper intoxication in maintenance dialysis has caused
A. a hard-water syndrome
B. acute hemolysis
C. erythrocytosis
D. progressive mental deterioration
E. peripheral neuropathy
REF. 7, p. 240

906. Persistently low blood pressure in an overhydrated dialysis patient with a normal heart shadow on x-ray is most likely due to
A. brown atrophy of the heat
B. Addison's disease
C. constrictive pericarditis
D. failed hypertension
E. amyloid
REF. 7, p. 271

907. Shortly after initiating a hemodialysis the patient complains of arm pain, followed by chest pain, dyspnea, and hypotension. This may be due to
A. incomplete rinsing of the dialyzer
B. too high dialysate calcium
C. too high dialysate magnesium
D. copper contamination
E. forgetting to give heparin
REF. 5, p. 857

908. Immediately after hemodialysis the most common acid-base abnormality is
A. metabolic acidosis
B. respiratory acidosis
C. metabolic alkalosis
D. respiratory alkalosis
E. mixed metabolic alkalosis and respiratory acidosis
REF. 5, p. 853

909. What factor is NOT included in the formula used for the calculation of dialysance?
A. Dialysate flow
B. Blood flow
C. Concentration gradient
D. Arterial concentration
E. Venous concentration
REF. 5, p. 839

10. PREGNANCY AND THE KIDNEY

DIRECTIONS: Each of the questions or incomplete statements below is followed by five suggested answers or completions. Select the one that is best in each case.

---

910. All of the following occur during pregnancy EXCEPT
   A. total body water increases
   B. blood volume decreases
   C. cardiac output increases
   D. renal blood flow increases
   E. GFR increases
   REF. 7, p. 1321

911. During pregnancy
   A. red cell mass increases, but less so than plasma volume
   B. cardiac output decreases
   C. peripheral resistance decreases
   D. vasodilation is evident clinically
   E. physiologic anemia reflects hemodilution
   REF. 7, p. 1321

912. During pregnancy
   A. average BUN is 19 mg/100 ml
   B. average serum creatinine is 0.5 mg/100 ml
   C. uric acid increases
   D. an increased serum bicarbonate level reflects compensation for metabolic alkalosis
   E. urinary amino acid levels are reduced
   REF. 8, pp. 472-474

913. The average BUN in pregnancy is
   A. 3 mg%
   B. 9 mg%
   C. 14 mg%
   D. 20 mg%
   E. 24 mg%
   REF. 7, p. 1323

914. Which of the following does NOT increase sodium reabsorption during pregnancy?
A. Increased filtration fraction
B. Aldosterone
C. Progesterone
D. Estrogens
E. Cortisol
REF. 7, p. 1321

915. The concentration of which of the following ions increases during pregnancy?
A. Calcium
B. Sulfate
C. Sodium
D. Bicarbonate
E. Chloride
REF. 5, p. 1386

916. Sodium retention in pregnancy is favored by
A. increased glomerular filtration rate
B. progesterone
C. aldosterone
D. decreased cardiac output
E. low serum proteins
REF. 7, p. 1321

917. The pedal edema in most pregnant women is due to
A. salt retention
B. hypoalbuminemia
C. increased capillary permeability
D. increased venous pressure
E. increased blood pressure
REF. 5, p. 1386

918. All of the following are true of edema of normal pregnancy EXCEPT
A. it affects about 80% of women
B. it tends to appear late in the day and clears overnight
C. it may be generalized, affecting the hands and face, in about 20% of women
D. it can be treated with moderate salt restriction and bed rest
E. diuretics are always contraindicated
REF. 7, p. 1386

919. Seizures during induction of labor with oxytocin drip of 5% dextrose/water are most likely due to
A. subarachnoid hemorrhage
B. cerebral thrombosis
C. water intoxication
D. hyperosmolarity
E. hyperglycemia
REF. 5, p. 1386

920. Asymptomatic bacteria of pregnancy is most likely to cause
A. anemia
B. prematurity
C. congenital abnormalities
D. pyelonephritis
E. toxemia
REF. 8, p. 488

921. A 20-year-old gravida 1 is found to have proteinuria with normal blood pressure and no edema in the first trimester; the likely cause is
A. toxemia
B. early essential hypertension
C. urinary tract infection
D. chronic glomerulonephritis
E. nephrosclerosis
REF. 8, p. 479

922. The most characteristic feature of preeclampsia is
A. immune-deposits of IgA
B. glomerular thrombosis
C. crescent formation
D. endotheliosis
E. cortical necrosis
REF. 7, p. 1339

923. Factors that predispose a woman to preeclampsia are all of the following EXCEPT
A. first pregnancy
B. tall, thin body build
C. multiple pregnancy
D. hydramnios
E. essential hypertension
REF. 7, p. 1342

924. Preeclampsia may result from all of the following predisposing factors EXCEPT
A. essential hypertension
B. coarctation of the aorta
C. unilateral renal artery disease
D. chronic glomerulonephritis
E. pyelonephritis
REF. 7, p. 1341

925. Preeclampsia may be prevented by
A. low-salt diet
B. diuretics
C. bed rest
D. high vitamin intake
E. restricted fluid intake
REF. 7, p. 1345

926. All of the following renal pathologic changes are seen in preeclampsia EXCEPT
A. glomerular endotheliosis
B. fibrin in endothelial cells
C. subendothelial deposits
D. increase in mesangial cells and matrix
E. granular deposits of immune complexes on the basement membrane
REF. 7, p. 1338

927. Renal abnormalities in toxemia include
A. low urine sodium
B. increased urate clearance
C. increased GFR
D. increased filtration fraction
E. hemodilution
REF. 5, p. 1382

928. Essential hypertension rather than toxemia of pregnancy is more likely if
A. the hypertension appears after 28 weeks
B. the patient is a primipara
C. proteinuria and edema are present
D. the serum uric acid is normal
E. the blood pressure was normal between pregnancies
REF. 8, p. 480

929. All of the following are found in preeclampsia EXCEPT
A. increased vascular reactivity to pressor agents
B. raised serum uric acid level
C. low serum lactate
D. intravascular coagulation
E. intensive ischemia
REF. 7, p. 480

930. Which of the following agents is most widely used in treating the hypertension of pregnancy?
A. Sodium nitroprusside
B. Hydralazine
C. Minoxidil
D. Captopril
E. Reserpine
REF. 7, p. 1345

931. In postpartum renal failure which of the following is LEAST likely to develop?
A. Hypertension
B. Thrombocytopenia
C. Fibrinoid necrosis
D. Microangiopathic hemolytic anemia
E. IgG deposits in glomeruli
REF. 7, p. 1333

932. Postpartum renal failure is characterized by the following clinical factors. Which of these is LEAST likely to be found in this setting?
A. Acute, severe, and usually irreversible renal failure beginning between 1 day and several months postpartum
B. The majority of patients have some complication of the pregnancy or delivery
C. A microangiopathic hemolytic anemia is present in all patients
D. Thrombocytopenia is present in most patients
E. Slowly developing hypertension and seizures are frequently associated phenomena
REF. 7, p. 1333

933. Reversal of toxemia after delivery is due to
A. loss of the placenta
B. loss of the fetus
C. decompression of the uterus
D. decompression of the ureter
E. loss of liquor amnii
REF. 10, p. 1794

934. Which of the following is LEAST characteristic of essential hypertension during pregnancy?
A. Rise in blood pressure during the second trimester
B. Increased incidence of toxemia
C. Increased incidence of abruptio placentae
D. Increased incidence of abortion
E. Increased incidence of prematurity
REF. 3, p. 980

935. A 20-year-old white gravida 1 in the third trimester of pregnancy is found to have proteinuria and hypertension. Measurement of which of the following substances would reveal a higher level than expected for an uncomplicated third trimester pregnancy?
A. Renin substrate
B. Plasma angiotensin II
C. Plasma aldosterone
D. Plasma renin activity
E. None of the above
REF. 7, p. 1337

936. Which of the following does NOT occur in normal pregnancy?
A. Increased cardiac output
B. Decreased plasma albumin concentration
C. Decreased uric acid clearance
D. Decreased serum creatinine level
E. Increased inulin clearance
REF. 8, p. 471

11. IMMUNOLOGY AND TRANSPLANTATION

DIRECTIONS: Each of the questions or incomplete statements below is followed by five suggested answers or completions. Select the one that is best in each case.

A. Immunology

937. Which of the following statements is NOT true concerning nephrotoxic serum nephritis (Masugi) ?
   A. Basement membrane antigen is injected into the animal to be studied
   B. An immediate episode of proteinuria
   C. An episode of proteinuria about 1 week after injection
   D. Proliferative changes in the glomerulus
   E. Fibrin is deposited in the glomerulus
   REF. 3, p. 334

938. Regarding experimental nephritis using autologous or heterologous tissue as antigen, which of the following statements is FALSE ?
   A. Deposits of IgG and B_1C globulin occur within the basement membrane
   B. Subepithelial deposits are usually found
   C. The antigen in Heymann nephritis is from the brush border of the proximal tubule
   D. Freund adjuvant is required in this model of nephritis
   E. All of the above statements are correct
   REF. 3, p. 309

939. Acute serum sickness is LEAST likely to cause
   A. necrotizing arteritis
   B. endothelial proliferation
   C. initial complexes that are soluble
   D. subendothelial deposits
   E. positive immunofluorescence to IgG
   REF. 3, p. 303

940. Which of the following factors are essential for development of acute serum sickness nephritis in the experimental animal?
A. Presence of complement
B. Polymorphonuclear cells
C. Large excess of antigen
D. Phagocytosis
E. None of the above
REF. 3, p. 307

941. Which of the following statements about acute serum sickness nephritis is FALSE?
A. The morphologic changes occur between 7 and 9 days after an injection of a foreign protein
B. Serum complement becomes depressed and gamma globulin is deposited in the glomerulus
C. The pathologic changes appear as the soluble complexes disappear from the circulation
D. Small antigen-antibody complexes formed in very great antigen excess have the most potent biologic activity
E. Hump-like deposits occur on the epithelial side of the basement membrane
REF. 7, p. 541

942. Concerning chronic serum sickness nephritis
A. it is produced by a single injection of foreign protein in slight antigen excess
B. large deposits of IgG and IgA are found in a subendothelial location
C. the lesion may resolve if large daily doses of antigen are injected
D. there is no evidence that complement is necessary in this model of nephritis
E. proliferation is conspicuously absent
REF. 7, p. 542

943. Experimentally, which is most important for precipitation of immune complexes?
A. Antigen less than equivalent to the amount of antibody
B. Moderate excess of antigen
C. Extreme excess of antigen
D. Nature of reacting components
E. Extreme excess of antibody
REF. 3, p. 333

944. Which of the following statements is NOT true of immune-complex-induced glomerulonephritis?
   A. Granular glomerular immunofluorescence for immunoglobulin and C3 is characteristic
   B. Lupus nephritis is caused by immune-complex mechanisms
   C. Hepatitis-B antigenemia may be associated with immune-complex glomerulonephritis
   D. Acute poststreptococcal glomerulonephritis is very similar to one-shot serum sickness in rabbits
   E. Immune-complex mechanisms have not been identified in tubulointerstitial diseases

   REF. 10, pp. 1246, 1311

945. The size of the immune complex depends on
   A. the size of antigen molecules and configuration of antigen determinants
   B. the firmness of antigen-antibody binding sites
   C. the immunoglobulin class of antibody
   D. interaction with the complement system
   E. all of the above

   REF. 3, p. 323

946. Deposition of immune complexes in the basement membrane has been found in the nephrotic syndrome associated with all of the following EXCEPT
   A. secondary syphilis
   B. malaria
   C. membranous glomerulopathy
   D. lupus nephritis
   E. minimal change nephritis

   REF. 10, p. 1293

947. Which of the following statements about diffuse glomerulonephritis in subacute bacterial endocarditis (SBE) is NOT true?
   A. It is usually found in the septicemic phase
   B. It occurs when bacterial antigen in the circulation is in relatively high concentration
   C. Concentration of antibody to pertinent antigen is relatively low
   D. Glomerulus contains complement
   E. It occurs only when antibody is in large excess relative to antigen concentration

   REF. 3, p. 585

948. In the acute phase of poststreptococcal glomerulonephritis immune complexes can be visualized by immunofluorescent reagents specific for
A. IgG and C3
B. IgA
C. IgM
D. C3 only
E. IgE
REF. 10, p. 1380

949. Which of the following statements concerning the role of the polymorphonuclear leukocytes (PMNL) in immune-complex disease is INCORRECT?
A. Depletion of circulating PMNL prevents the development of foreign protein nephritis
B. In acute membranous glomerulonephritis, the degree of PMNL infiltrates does not correlate with the degree of glomerular damage
C. In lupus mesangiopathic glomerulonephritis, PMNL are usually inconspicuous
D. In membranous glomerulopathy progressive damage to the glomerular basement membrane may occur without significant PMNL infiltrate
E. PMNL are not usually found in the vicinity of immune-complex deposits
REF. 3, p. 342

950. Systemic infection associated with immune-deposit nephritis is LEAST likely in which of the following conditions?
A. A 5-year-old child with heavy proteinuria, edema, lipiduria, and absence of hypertension
B. The development of nephrotic syndrome in an East-African man who has had recurrent episodes of fever and chills
C. Hematuria and edema in a 20-year-old woman with a nonpruritic rash, most marked on the palms and soles
D. Following surgery to correct obstructive hydrocephalus
E. Proteinuria and edema in a heroin addict
REF. 3, p. 347

951. Immune deposits of B_1C and IgG have been observed in all of the following EXCEPT
A. Henoch-Schönlein nephritis
B. Alport's syndrome
C. membranous glomerulonephritis
D. renal vein thrombosis
E. renal homograft rejection
REF. 7, p. 554

952. Immunofluorescence in Henoch-Schonlein nephritis normally occurs at the
A. tubule basement membrane
B. capillary loops
C. intraluminal sites
D. mesangium
E. none of the above
REF. 3, p. 748

953. Which of the following statements is FALSE concerning the complement system?
A. Activation (cleavage) of C3 is common to both the classic and the alternative pathways
B. Classic pathway activation proceeds through C1, C4, C2, in that order
C. In the alternative pathway various substances may cleave C3 by-passing C1, C4, C2
D. Immune complexes of antigen and IgG can activate C1 by binding to its subunit C1q
E. Once C3 is cleaved, the membrane attack mechanism is activated via C4
REF. 10, p. 1239

954. The biologic consequences of complement activation include all but which of the following?
A. Immune adherence
B. Polymorphonuclear chemotaxis
C. Increased capillary permeability from release of anaphylatoxins
D. Cellular lysis
E. Decreased phagocytosis
REF. 10, p. 1240

955. Regarding the assembly of the recognition and activator units in the classic complement pathway, which of the following statements is FALSE?
A. The C1 complex is formed of three different kinds of proteins
B. C1q binds on the antibodies present on cell surfaces
C. C1q deficiency conditions resembly systemic lupus erythematosus
D. C1s cleave C2 and C4 and these fragments form C3 convertase
E. C3 convertase cleaves C3 and the fragments C4b, 2a, 3b form C6
REF. 10, p. 1240

956. Which of the following statements is FALSE concerning anti-GBM antibody nephritis?
A. There is a linear immunofluorescence of IgG
B. Glomerular immunofluorescence for C3 is absent in 25 to 30% of the cases
C. Absence of C3 immunofluorescence indicates a better prognosis
D. Often there is a linear fluorescence for IgG around the tubular basement membrane
E. The picture is usually one of rapidly progressive, proliferative, necrotizing, and crescentic glomerulonephritis
REF. 10, p. 1260

957. Which of the following statements is NOT true of anti-GBM glomerulonephritis?
A. An antecedent flu-like illness is common
B. Some patients have had antecedent exposure to hydrocarbon solvent inhalation
C. Linear GBM fluorescence for IgG is found only in Goodpasture's syndrome
D. Anti-GBM antibodies can be detected in over half the cases by indirect immunofluorescence
E. Materials cross-reactive with GBM are present in normal urine, and accumulate in the serum after nephrectomy
REF. 10, p. 1256

958. The diagnosis of human antibasement glomerulonephritis should NOT be made by
A. the presence of a linear deposition of immunoglobulin in the glomerular wall
B. the presence of circulating antibasement antibodies after nephrectomy
C. electron microscopy combined with immunofluorescence
D. serologic tests
E. light microscopy alone
REF. 10, p. 1256

959. In human anti-GBM antibody glomerulonephritis after bilateral nephrectomy, anti-GBM antibodies in the serum
A. usually decrease markedly
B. usually increase and stay elevated for many years
C. do not change
D. usually deposit in extrarenal sites
E. are of no significance in further management before and after transplantation
REF. 3, p. 775

960. Membranous glomerulopathy may be distinguished best from minimal change disease (lipoid nephrosis) by
A. light microscope study
B. immunofluorescent study
C. volume of 24-hr urine output
D. 24-hr urine for protein electrophoresis
E. serum complement level
REF. 3, p. 348

961. Membranoproliferative glomerulonephritis and poststreptococcal glomerulonephritis may best be differentiated by
A. light microscopy and the mesangial cell proliferation
B. immunofluorescent study and the character of immunoglobulin deposition
C. electron microscopic study and the relation of electron-dense deposits to the basement membrane
D. the presence of hypocomplementemia in the early stages of the disease
E. lobular pattern found in membranoproliferative glomerulonephritis
REF. 3, p. 749

962. Which is the predominant type immunoglobulin present in the mesangium in mesangiopathic glomerulonephritis associated with benign essential hematuria?
A. IgG
B. IgA
C. IgE
D. IgM
E. C3 complement
REF. 10, p. 1400

963. Which of the following antibodies is most significant in the pathogenesis of lupus nephritis?
A. Anti-RNA protein
B. Antiextractable nuclear antigen (ENA)
C. Anti-DNA
D. Antimitochondrial antibodies
E. Antibasement antibody
REF. 10, p. 1495

964. Cytotoxic antibodies can be induced by all of the following EXCEPT
A. blood transfusion
B. pregnancies
C. infection
D. previous allograft
E. hemoglobin infusion
REF. 7, p. 470

965. Cytotoxic antibodies are most common in
A. multiparous women
B. adolescents
C. adult males
D. nonparous females
E. multiparous women with a history of blood transfusions
REF. 7, p. 470

966. Immunofluoresence in rapidly progressive glomerulonephritis may show all of the following EXCEPT
A. linear staining
B. IgG staining
C. C3 staining
D. IgM staining
E. any of the above may be present
REF. 3, p. 453

967. Which of the following is usually NOT an immunofluorescent feature of proliferative lupus glomerulonephritis?
A. Linear IgG deposition
B. Patchy IgG deposition
C. Granular C3 deposition
D. Fibrinogen deposition
E. IgM deposition
REF. 3, p. 863

968. Linear immunofluorescence for gamma globulin and B_1C globulin along the basement membrane of the glomerulus is most likely to be seen in
A. lupus nephritis
B. Goodpasture's syndrome
C. Henoch-Schönlein purpura
D. polyarteritis nodosa
E. thrombotic thrombocytopenic purpura
REF. 3, p. 775

969. The generally-found immunofluorescent stain in hemolytic uremic syndrome is
A. fibrinogen
B. IgG
C. IgA
D. IgM
E. complement
REF. 3, p. 923

B. Transplantation

970. In the cell destruction phase of transplant rejection immunology, which of the following systems is involved?
A. Effector T cells
B. Macrophages
C. Antibody-dependent cell-mediated cytolysis
D. Humoral antibodies
E. All of the above
REF. 6, p. 1471

971. The first cell to infiltrate an allograft following implantation is
A. T lymphocyte
B. B lymphocyte
C. polymorph
D. macrophage
E. eosinophil
REF. 3, p. 1471

972. The cell causing a humoral response to an allograft is the
   A. regional large lymphocyte
   B. plasma cell
   C. T lymphocyte
   D. macrophage invading the graft
   E. basophil
   REF. 3, p. 1470

973. The first abnormality to appear when a transplanted kidney begins to reject is reduction in
   A. effective renal blood flow
   B. total renal blood flow
   C. glomerular filtration rate
   D. filtration fraction
   E. T_mPAH
   REF. 3, p. 1462

974. Genes identified on chromosome 6 that play a role in transplant rejection include all of the following EXCEPT
   A. HLA complex
   B. Ir
   C. P-erythrocyte antigen
   D. LD system governing mixed lymphocyte culture reactions
   E. antinuclear antigens
   REF. 10, p. 2554

975. Which of the following tests most reliably indicates prolonged cadaveric graft survival before surgery?
   A. Lymphocytotoxicity test
   B. Mixed lymphocyte culture
   C. Leukoagglutination test
   D. Complement fixation test
   E. ABO blood group test
   REF. 10, p. 2579

976. Which of the following does NOT occur during acute rejection?
   A. Inhibition of sheep erythrocyte rosettes
   B. Inhibition of recipient leukocyte migration to donor antigen
   C. Increased number of peripheral lymphoblasts
   D. Falling platelet count
   E. Fall in the level of IgM
   REF. 10, p. 2583

977. The initiating event in hyperacute rejection is
   A. platelet aggregation
   B. fibrinogen activation
   C. leukocyte margination
   D. antigen binding to endothelium of kidney
   E. antibody binding to endothelium of kidney
   REF. 3, p. 1473

978. Transplantation should NOT be carried out on
   A. cadaver donor with two antigen HLA matching
   B. cadaver donor with no HLA matching
   C. related donor with four HLA matching and a different blood group
   D. recipient with a history of blood transfusion in the past
   E. sibling with three HLA matching and the same blood group
   REF. 10, p. 2561

979. A 32-year-old male had a cadaveric transplantation about 12 weeks ago and for the last 7 days his blood pressure was found to be 180/120 mmHg. He is on prednisone 20 mg/day. He should
   A. be treated with IV prednisolone 1 g/day
   B. have emergency arteriography
   C. have prednisone dose reduced to 5 mg/day
   D. have prednisone stopped and IV furosemide (Lasix) 40 mg given
   E. have prednisone maintained in the same dose and azathioprine increased
   REF. 10, p. 2634

980. Hyperacute rejection occurring within hours of a transplant is best prevented by
   A. high-dose intravenous prednisone
   B. intraarterial prednisone and heparin
   C. antilymphocytic globulin
   D. careful preoperative screening for cytotoxic antibodies
   E. plasmapheresis
   REF. 10, p. 2633

981. In the early posttransplant phase following a living related donor transplant
   A. urinary calcium excretion is increased
   B. phosphaturia occurs
   C. patients develop severe hypocalcemia
   D. decreased bone reabsorption occurs
   E. none of the above
   REF. 10, p. 2648

982. The immunosuppressive effects of corticosteroids are due to all of the following EXCEPT
   A. karyorrhexis of T cells
   B. margination of leukocytes
   C. reduced antibody synthesis
   D. inhibition of granulocyte migration
   E. inhibition of chemotaxis of granulocytes
   REF. 10, p. 2626

983. Which of the following regarding posttransplantation pancreatitis is FALSE?
   A. Occurs in 5-15% of patients
   B. May be caused by immunological mechanisms
   C. Carries a 50% mortality
   D. Steroids may be responsible
   E. Is due to cyclosporin
   REF. 10, p. 2650

984. Recurrence of the underlying renal disease after transplantation is LEAST likely with which of the following?
   A. Medullary cystic disease
   B. Amyloidosis
   C. Dense-deposit disease
   D. Oxalosis
   E. Goodpasture's syndrome
   REF. 10, p. 2619

985. A transplant performed between two nonidentical twins is termed
   A. an allograft
   B. a xenograft
   C. an isograft
   D. a syngeneic graft
   E. a heterograph
   REF. 10, p. 2545

986. A potential transplant recipient is found to have, on tissue typing, A_2 B_{18}/A_{11} B_{13}. He has two siblings of the same blood type. Sibling #1 is A_2 B_{13}/A_x B_8 and sibling #2 is A_2 B_{18}/A_x B_8 and all have negative cross-matches. In selecting a donor
A. sibling #1 should be used
B. sibling #2 should be used
C. neither sibling is suitable
D. an MLC test should be done to pick the best donor
E. there has been an error in the tissue typing
REF. 7, p. 467

In performing an MLC test using mitomycin-C-treated cells (designated by $_m$) between two related donors (D_1 and D_2) and a recipient (R) as well as an unrelated control (C) the following results are obtained on thymidine incorporation testing.

R	3695	$R+R_m$	3800	D_2+R_m	61000
Rm	98	$R+D_1$	28090	D_1+C_m	95000
D_1	2695	$R+D_{1m}$	4500	D_2+C_m	91000
D_{1m}	150	$R+D_2$	65000		
D_2	2550	$R+D_{2m}$	39000		
D_{2m}	200	R+C	72000		
C	3100	$R+C_m$	85000		
C_m	175	D_1+R_m	49500		

987. The most suitable donor is
A. donor 1
B. donor 2
C. control
D. any of the above are equally suitable
E. none of the above should be used
REF. 7, p. 468.

988. In potential transplant recipients, the cross-match cytotoxic reaction consists of which of the following reactions?
A. Donor serum and recipient lymphocytes
B. Donor lymphocytes and recipient serum
C. Donor serum and recipient serum
D. Donor lymphocytes and recipient lymphocytes
E. All of the above
REF. 7, p. 470

989. Patients with which of the following two diseases are most suitable renal transplant candidates?
A. Advanced obstructive lung disease
B. Fabry's disease
C. Oxalosis
D. Cysteinosis
E. Membranous nephropathy
REF. 7, p. 473

990. Six weeks following renal transplant, a patient develops azotemia and oliguria and low-grade fever; a renal biospy reveals fibrin deposition and necrosis in the glomeruli and small vessels as well as polymorph infiltrate in the glomerulus. What type of rejection does this patient have?
A. Accelerated
B. Acute
C. Chronic
D. Hyperacute
E. None of above
REF. 7, p. 490

991. Which of the following diseases would most likely recur following renal transplantation?
A. Posterior urethral valves
B. Alport's syndrome
C. Primary oxalosis
D. Lupus erythematosus
E. Cancer with nonrecurrence in 5 years
REF. 10, p. 2620

992. The most common tumor in transplant recipients is
A. Kaposi's sarcoma
B. carcinoma of cervix
C. lymphomas
D. skin cancers
E. bronchogenic carcinoma
REF. 10, p. 2642

993. Which of the following tumors is LEAST common following renal transplantation?
A. Reticulum cell sarcoma
B. Carcinoma of lung
C. Carcinoma of cervix
D. Basal cell carcinoma of lip
E. Squamous cell carcinoma of lip
REF. 7, p. 502

994. Three weeks after renal transplant a patient suddenly develops pain and swelling over his graft and goes into shock; the most likely diagnosis is
A. acute rejection
B. acute arterial occlusion
C. kidney rupture
D. lymphocele
E. recurrent glomerulonephritis
REF. 3, p. 1517

995. In a transplant recipient who develops oliguria, which of the following tests is most helpful in distinguishing a non-viable kidney from acute tubular necrosis?
A. Serum creatinine
B. BUN
C. I^{131} hyppurate scan
D. Urine osmolality
E. Urine sodium
REF. 10, p. 2633

996. In hyperacute rejection the first abnormality to occur is
A. proliferation of recipient lymphocytes
B. coating of graft vessel with antibody
C. fibrinogen activation
D. platelet aggregation
E. vascular thrombosis
REF. 3, p. 1479

997. In acute humeral rejection the main cell in the renal interstitium is
A. T lymphocytes
B. B lymphocytes
C. lymphoblasts
D. plasma cells
E. macrophages
REF. 3, p. 1487

998. The best way to monitor for azothioprine toxicity is by
A. serum bilirubin
B. serum alkaline phosphate
C. serum creatinine
D. hemoglobin
E. peripheral leukocyte count
REF. 10, p. 2626

999. Cyclosporin A possesses all but which one of the following features?
A. Damages lymphoblasts
B. Damages polymorphs
C. Nephrotoxic
D. Hepatoxic
E. Is a fungal metabolite
REF. 10, p. 2631

1000. The glomerular lesion most suggestive of transplant rejection is
A. IgA deposits in mesangium
B. type I membranoproliferative glomerulonephritis
C. subepithelial deposits
D. minimal change disease
E. none of the above
REF. 10, p. 2637

1001. The most common infection in the transplant recipient is
A. Pneumocystic carinii
B. listeria meningitis
C. pneumococcal pneumonia
D. influenza
E. cytomegalovirus
REF. 10, p. 2624

EXPLANATORY ANSWERS

The authors have made every effort to thoroughly verify the answers to the questions which appear on the preceding pages. However, as in any text, some inaccuracies and ambiguities may occur; therefore, if in doubt, please consult your references.

The Publisher

---

1. PHYSIOLOGY

1. (A) Some 15% of nephrons have long loops of Henle extending deep into the medulla and able to reabsorb sodium efficiently.

2. (D) Infusion of saline or water will increase ascites and edema whereas albumin and dextran will raise the plasma oncotic pressure and cause a shift of extracellular fluid into the plasma. Ultimately, however, the albumin will enter the peritoneal cavity and the dextran will be lost in the urine.

3. (E) Amino acid levels are often markedly increased in lactic acidosis.

4. (B) NH_3 production is increased in all segments of the nephron during acidosis. During prolonged acidosis there is additional adaptive increase in phosphate-dependent glutaminase activity in the proximal convoluted tubule.

5. (D) Dopamine acts on a specific vascular receptor site and phenothiazines deplete dopamine stores.

6. (B) In alcoholic ketoacidosis the beta-hydroxybutyrate to acetoacetate ratio in plasma is increased.

7. (B) Eighty percent of the ketone bodies are beta-hydroxybutyrate.

8. (B) Since actinomycin D inhibits protein synthesis, increase in enzyme activity in its presence is the result of activation of existing enzyme and/or decrease in decay of enzyme rather than the synthesis of new enzyme protein.

9. (B) With osmotic diuresis, there is an obligatory water loss with the nonreabsorbed solutes.

10. (A) All parenteral feeding regimens are based on amino acids.

11. (A) Glomerular filtration and renal plasma flow increase proportionately.

12. (C) Daily exercise of 100 minutes for 10 days generally provides optimum adaptation.

13. (C) Antidiuretic hormone is increased because of hyperosmolality, hypovolemia, and a direct action of heat on the pituitary.

14. (D) Because of hypercatabolism, the blood urea level is proportionately elevated.

15. (C) The cell swells because of the reduced active transport of sodium out of the cell.

16. (E) The total body potassium is usually normal in hypothyroidism.

17. (D) The colon actively secretes bicarbonate and conserves sodium.

18. (A) In mild stress renal blood flow decreases minimally, with no change in glomerular filtration, but in severe stress renal blood flow decreases markedly and filtration rate may remain constant or decrease to a lesser extent so that the filtration fraction increases.

19. (E) Inulin clearance measures glomerular filtration rate.

20. (D) The glomerular filtration rate and renal blood flow in a 90-year-old man are reduced by 50%.

21. (C) Vasopressin in physiologic doses has no effect on renal blood flow.

22. (B) Cold increases renal blood flow.

23. (E) Ten percent of basement membrane is carbohydrate containing disaccharides and heteropolysaccharides.

24. (C) Ferritin is a large particle with a high molecular weight, and is concentrated on the endothelial side of the basement membrane.

25. (E) Horseradish peroxidase, with a molecular weight of 40,000, rapidly enters the urinary space, whereas myeloperoxidase with a molecular weight of 160,000 is held up at the slit pores. Likewise, albumin is held up at the epithelial slit pores.

26. (C) In nephrosclerosis the renal blood flow is depressed more than the glomerular filtration rate, so that the filtration fraction is increased.

27. (A) Horseradish peroxidase and myeloperoxidase have been shown to be taken up by mesangial cells.

28. (E) Proteinuria may be induced in normal subjects by injection of epinephrine, exercise, or by renal ischemia resulting from dehydration, surgery, hemorrhage, or salt depletion.

29. (E) The tubular lumen of the ascending limb is electrically positive with respect to peritubular fluid, and the potential is eliminated by adding oubain or by substituting sulfate for chloride in the perfusion fluids.

30. (D) The descending limb is water permeable and the ascending limb is solute permeable.

31. (C) Urine is finally concentrated in the collecting duct by reabsorption of water.

32. (B) Active chloride transport is responsible for positive voltage in the lumen

33. (C) At the tip of the loop of Henle, the tubular and interstitial fluids are nearly isosmolar.

34. (A-1) Urine is an ultrafiltrate of plasma.
(B-1) Reabsorption in the proximal tubule is isosmotic.

(C-3) Sodium enters the tubule from a hypertonic interstitium.
(D-2) Sodium is actively reabsorbed; however the membrane is impermeable to water.

35. (B) The proximal tubular fluid is isosmotic with plasma in a variety of conditions in which the final urine is hypotonic or hypertonic.

36. (B) Acute contraction of the extracellular fluid volume or blood volume causes increased reabsorption of Na from proximal tubule; whereas aldosterone has a powerful effect on Na reabsorption in the distal tubule.

37. (D) The final urinary content of the other substances is contributed mainly by tubular secretion.

38. (E) Acidification increases the ionization of weak bases and thus decreases nonionic back diffusion from the renal tubule.

39. (B) Carrier-mediated secretion is specific for cations as well as amino acids and monosaccharides.

40. (E) Probenecid blocks the secretion of penicillin since both involve the same pump.

41. (D) During potassium depletion, as well as during the administration of acetazolamide, and in renal tubular acidosis, the intracellular pH is lowered and citrate excretion rate is diminished.

42. (C) TmPAH is the point beyond which no further increment in tubular secretion occurs.

43. (A) There is increased delivery of hypotonic fluid from the loop of Henle.

44. (B) Free water is formed as a result of active sodium and chloride reabsorption at the diluting sites in the ascending limb of the loop of Henle.

45. (D) Weak acids diffuse out of the tubular lumen more rapidly in the presence of excess H+; this suppresses the dissociation of the acid.

46. (E) Injection of albumin into the peritubular space increases

active reabsorption much more than passive reabsorption, as shown by the experimental addition of cyanide.

47. (B) Vasopressin is bound to receptors on the basolateral surface of the tubule, causing increased permeability of the luminal surface to water.

48. (D) Free water clearance represents urine volume minus osmolar clearance, and is negative when the urine is concentrated.

49. (A) Urea is accounted for in the calculation of the estimated plasma osmolality.

50. (D) The onset of diabetes insipidus is often sudden, whereas that of compulsive polydypsia is likely to be less well defined.

51. (E) Extracellular volume contraction increases proximal tubular reabsorption and decreases sodium delivery to the diluting sites.

52. (A) Calcium inhibits adenylate cyclase and the binding of vasopressin to its receptors.

53. (E) All of the choices except penicillin may alter the function of the distal tubule or collecting duct and produce nephrogenic diabetes insipidus.

54. (C) Deuterium oxide, an isotope of water, is evenly distributed throughout the body water.

55. (B) Phosphodiesterase inactivates cyclic AMP.

56. (A) Because adipose tissue contains less water than lean tissue, the percentage of body water is lowest in an obese person.

57. (B) In water diuresis, the osmolality of the urine of man may be only one-tenth or less that of blood plasma.

58. (E) Furosemide increases sodium and calcium excretion; chronic chlorothiazide therapy increases sodium excretion and decreases calcium excretion; parathormone causes hypercalciuria but does not change sodium excretion. Desoxycorticosterone acutely causes sodium retention but no

change in calcium excretion; chronically there is hypercalciuria and sodium excretion rises to normal levels.

59. (B) At high rates of vasopressin (Pitressin) infusion, changes in urine flow are less striking than the U/P creatinine ratio, which shows a graded response.

60. (A) Water is lost proportionately from all body spaces.

61. (B) The reflexes are increased.

62. (B) Sodium exists in the same concentration in the interstitial fluid as in plasma; and as interstitial fluid is greater than plasma, total sodium in interstitial fluid is greater.

63. (C) About one-half of the total body sodium is in the extracellular space. The other half is intracellular most of which is in bone.

64. (D) Albumin may cause contraction of the interstitial fluid compartment, and may cause sodium retention.

65. (E) Estrogens cause salt retention.

66. (D) The excretion of creatinine is determined mainly by its plasma level.

67. (C) The ascending limb is impermeable to water.

68. (A) Infusion of iso-oncotic albumin produces water diuresis.

69. (E) Phenytoin inhibits ADH release.

70. (C) Antidiuretic hormone stimulates active sodium transport across certain tissues.

71. (E) Antidiuretic hormone activates adenylcyclase, which converts adenosine triphosphate to 3'5'-adenosine monophosphate.

72. (E) The release of ADH is regulated by osmoreceptors. Vasopressin is an octapeptide which contains arginine in man and lysine in the pig.

73. (B) Urea causes no change in intracellular volume because it is diffusible.

74. (A) Morphine stimulates antidiuretic hormone release.

75. (D) Alcohol inhibits release of antidiuretic hormone.

76. (E) In bronchogenic carcinoma, the release of ADH is "inappropriate."

77. (D) Chlorpropamide may act in the kidney by inhibiting prostaglandin synthesis

78. (C) Aldosterone potentiates the effect of antidiuretic hormone, probably by inhibiting phosphodiesterase.

79. (A) High concentrations of demeclocycline inhibit cyclic AMP production and cyclic AMP action in the toad bladder. Its point of action in man has not been established.

80. (B) Isoproterenol is a beta-adrenergic agent, and as such has an antidiuretic effect.

81. (C) Mineralocorticoid deficiency causes a negative sodium balance in patients with Addison's disease; but cortisone deficiency also promotes hyponatremia by other mechanisms.

82. (D) Some investigators have found that antidiuretic hormone levels are inappropriately high in hypothyroidism.

83. (C) Effective plasma volume is decreased in cardiac failure.

84. (D) Decreased proximal sodium reabsorption is a response to plasma volume expansion.

85. (C) Lithium produces nephrogenic diabetes insipidus by inhibiting vasopressin mediated increases in cyclic AMP.

86. (C) Phenytoin causes a diuresis probably by inhibiting antidiuretic hormone release. The mechanism of acetohexamide induced diuresis is not known.

87. (E) The free water clearance represents sodium reabsorption at dilution sites, provided it is assumed that no further water is reabsorbed in the collecting duct. During water diuresis the free water clearance may easily reach 10 to 15 ml/min.

88. (A) Urine is less than maximally dilute but urine osmolality may be less than that of serum. On a normal Na intake patients with SIADH will have high urine Na.

89. (D) Urea is freely permeable, and the "effective" solute load is not increased in the plasma.

90. (E) Renal artery constriction increases sodium reabsorption.

91. (C) Evidence that Na transport is an active process comes from the finding of a linear relationship between renal oxygen consumption and Na reabsorption, so that about 20 to 30 mEq of Na are reabsorbed per mole of oxygen.

92. (B) Hyperglycemia normally tends to lower serum sodium concentration; hypernatremia indicates profound water loss, in excess of sodium and other ions.

93. (B) Water and salt retention frequently occur during refeeding; the edema can be minimized by a low-sodium diet. Eventually, a spontaneous diuresis occurs.

94. (C) The amount of water in a given volume of plasma is reduced, hence the "pseudohyponatremia."

95. (C) Such patients tolerate salt loads well.

96. (B) In water deprivation there is contraction of the extracellular fluid and sodium retention.

97. (C) Sodium chloride acts as an osmotic diuretic so that the urine becomes more dilute.

98. (C) In alkalosis potassium moves into the cells in exchange for hydrogen ion.

99. (E) In states of potassium depletion potassium reabsorption continues in the distal tubule and collecting duct, and very small amounts only are excreted in the urine.

100. (B) In the distal tubule potassium secretion is not dependent on a 1:1 exchange with sodium, and usually changes in parallel with hydrogen ion secretion.

101. (A) Decreased sodium delivery to the distal tubule decreases K^+ secretion, the flow rate of tubular fluid being

an important modulator of K+ transport at this site.

102. (C) Filtered potassium is almost completely reabsorbed by the proximal tubule and ascending loop of Henle, and only 5 - 10% reaches the distal tubule.

103. (B) An inability to conserve phosphate in some patients with hypokalemia may cause severe hypophosphatemia.

104. (B) Potassium deficiency impairs renal ability to conserve sodium.

105. (A) Reversibility of vacuolation by potassium repletion has been established.

106. (A) Potassium deficiency is most commonly associated with impairment of urinary concentration.

107. (E) K deficiency can result in hypomagnesemia.

108. (D) Decreased potassium excretion occurs as a consequence of hypoaldosteronism, with decreased potassium secretion in the distal convoluted tubule.

109. (E) Hypoaldosteronism is probably present; salt and mineralocorticosteroids may help.

110. (A) Destruction of leukocytes and platelets causes a pseudohyperkalemia which can be diagnosed by measuring potassium in plasma rather than in serum. The other features are characteristic of the hypokalemia occasionally seen in leukemia.

111. (C) A low aldosterone level leads to acidosis as well as hyperkalemia.

112. (A) If there is acute extracellular hyperkalemia with little change in intracellular potassium the resting membrane potential is reduced.

113. (C) The QT (or rather the QU) interval tends to be prolonged in hypokalemia.

114. (C) Phosphate is handled mainly by proximal tubular reabsorption; distal tubular reabsorption plays a relatively minor role.

115. (B) Hypomagnesemia causes phosphaturia, even in the absence of parathormone.

116. (D) Only parathormone is clearly important in homeostatic regulation of renal phosphate excretion.

117. (B) Phosphate may disappear from the urine as the blood level falls.

118. (B) Calcium inhibits parathormone secretion and decreases phosphate excretion; the others interfere with phosphate reabsorption in the proximal tubule.

119. (D) Phlorizin augments the phosphate Tm and increases phosphate reabsorption by eradicating the competition for glucose reabsorption.

120. (E) Magnesium inhibits parathyroid activity and results in phosphate reabsorption by the proximal tubule

121. (B) Parathormone enhances distal tubular reabsorption of calcium, but the overall effect may be hypercalciuria because of the increased filtered load of calcium.

122. (E) Phosphate loading usually causes a decrease in urinary calcium by raising the solubility product in the blood.

123. (B) Stop-flow experiments indicate that accelerated reabsorption of calcium as a result of parathormone infusion takes place in the distal tubule.

124. (E) Hypercalciuria with metabolic acidosis is due to distal nephron stimulation.

125. (E) Hypercalciuria is augmented with combined elevated perfusion pressure and renal vasodilatation but aortic constriction abolishes the calciuric effects of vasodilatation.

126. (C) In the distal tubule calcium reabsorption is increased by parathormone and thiazides, and is dissociated from sodium reabsorption.

127. (E) Parathyroid hormone has a dual effect on the renal tubule. The net effect usually is to decrease calcium excretion.

128. (D) Acute calcium loads have been reported to increase the renal excretion of magnesium, possibly through competition by both divalent cations for a common reabsorption mechanism.

129. (D) Measuring total parathormone levels is useful in diagnosing hyperparathyroidism.

130. (D) Chronic administration of acetazolamide produces metabolic acidosis with hypercalciuria; chronic administration of thiazides produces hypocalciuria as a result of volume contraction and potentiation of parathormone on distal nephron effects. Osmotic diuretics also are calciuric.

131. (D) Glucocorticords have no direct effect on phosphate transport.

132. (D) Some 80% of magnesium is reabsorbed distally, whereas the other ions are reabsorbed to a greater extent in the proximal tubule.

133. (D) In dogs and rats parathormone has been shown to reduce both calcium and magnesium excretion.

134. (A) Magnesium's ability to cause neurodepression has been applied to the treatment of preeclampsia and eclampsia.

135. (C) Magnesium levels may be increased in uremia but can be low in other states mentioned.

136. (A) Tubular reabsorption equals the filtered load (glomerular filtration times plasma level) minus the amount excreted in the urine per unit time.

137. (A) Titratable acid represents the buffering capacity of the urine and the pH of the final urine represents the consumption of this buffer.

138. (D) Sulfate is not a buffer.

139. (C) The major fraction of an acute acid load is neutralized by buffers of cells and bone.

140. (A) The body is limited in its ability to rapidly buffer an acute increase of CO_2.

141. (B) One millimole of any gas occupies this volume.

142. (B) Rapid normalization of plasma bicarbonate concentration in metabolic acidosis will result in life-threatening metabolic and respiratory alkalosis as hyperventilation continues and organic anions are converted to bicarbonate.

143. (B) It hydrolyzes carbon dioxide to form carbonic acid.

144. (C) In hypokalemia there is extracellular alkalosis, intracellular acidosis, acid urine, and increased bicarbonate reabsorption.

145. (B) Infusion of potassium salts results in intracellular alkalosis, extracellular acidosis, and alkaline urine.

146. (E) Aldosterone encances H+ secretion, but this may depend on a concomitant potassium deficiency.

147. (D) Hydrogen ion secretion is active and is enhanced by carbonic anhydrase.

148. (B) Bicarbonate is not truly Tm-dependent and reabsorption is dependent on carbonic anhydrase and blocked by acetazolamide.

149. (D) During alkalosis, plasma citrate increases, causing a fall in ionized calcium which contributes to stimulation of parathormone secretion. PTH inhibits carbonic anhydrase activity via cyclic AMP.

150. (B) Intracellular pH regulates citrate reabsorption by influencing citrate entry across the luminal membrane of the tubule cell through a mechanism which is not related to the effect of intracellular fluid pH on citrate metabolism or to the citrate in renal tubule cells.

151. (B) Metabolic alkalosis stimulates conversion of glucose to lactate by the renal medulla and cortex.

152. (B) NH_3 is uncharged, lipid soluble, penetrates the cell membrane readily, and is a base.

153. (A) Potassium depletion increases ammonium excretion because the urine becomes alkaline, and NH_3 diffuses into the tubular lumen.

154. (C) Ammonia is more alkaline than the blood pH, so that titration will not free hydrogen ion.

155. (E) Titratable acidity is decreased in all these conditions.

156. (A) From the depressant effect of drugs and incisional pains which limit breathing, respiratory acidosis occurs after surgery.

157. (A) There is increased PCO_2, which crosses into CSF.

158. (C) In renal tubular acidosis there is usually a hyperchloremic acidosis with normal anion gap.

159. (A) A raised PCO_2 increases hydrogen ion excretion.

160. (D) The acids responsible for paraldehyde-induced metabolic acidosis have not been identified.

161. (D) The bicarbonate deficit equals 50% of body weight multiplied by the difference between the desired and actual bicarbonate blood level.

162. (C) In chronic renal failure the ability to acidify urine maximally is preserved.

163. (B) In acute respiratory acidosis 97% of the buffering mechanism is cellular.

164. (D) Acid retained in patients with renal disease is buffered by bone.

165. (A) Final correction of metabolic acidosis induced by acid infusion depends on renal excretion of acid.

166. (B) In acute respiratory alkalosis the extracellular stores of sodium, potassium, and bicarbonate decrease, and those of chloride and lactate increase.

167. (D) Plasma proteins represent the sole extracellular buffer in acute respiratory alkalosis. They account for 1% of the total buffering, the rest being intracellular.

168. (C) There is chloride depletion due to bicarbonate retention.

169. (B) Chloride administration will correct the alkalosis as it results from chloride depletion.

170. (D) Diuretic treated patients with cor pulmonale may have a mixed respiratory acidosis and metabolic alkalosis; in the other conditions a respiratory alkalosis may occur.

171. (C) The renal response to respiratory alkalosis is bicarbonate excretion.

172. (D) Acetazolamide causes metabolic acidosis.

173. (E) Carbon dioxide inspiration causes respiratory acidosis.

174. (B) The respiratory response to metabolic alkalosis is hypoventilation.

175. (D) Acid and chloride losses are consequences of nasogastric suction.

176. (C) The PCO_2 rises by 0. 6 mmHg for each millimole of bicarbonate.

177. (B) There is obligatory sodium reabsorption in the distal tubule resulting in increased tubular secretion of potassium.

178. (A) Diarrhea causes metabolic acidosis because of excessive bicarbonate loss.

179. (C) In pure metabolic acidosis each millimole fall in bicarbonate is associated with a 1. 2 mmHg fall in PCO_2.

180. (B) Hypoventilation of such a severe degree secondary to metabolic alkalosis is unlikely.

181. (E) In a pure respiratory alkalosis the PCO_2 would be lower.

182. (C) Hyperchloremic acidosis with a normal "anion gap" is most likely due to severe diarrhea.

183. (C) This pattern shows respiratory alkalosis and persistent hyperventilation.

184. (A) In acute respiratory acidosis the bicarbonate would not rise this high; the values fall within the 95% confidence band for chronic respiratory acidosis.

185. (B) The anion gap increases to some extent in metabolic alkalosis (from lactate). It decreases in bromide intoxication and some hyperglobulinemic states.

186. (D) The patient has respiratory acidosis from his lung disease and metabolic alkalosis from diuretics.

187. (E) About 12 g of nitrogen are excreted daily as uric acid, creatinine, urea, amino acids, and ammonia.

188. (B) Arginase splits arginine to urea and L-ornithine.

189. (A) A low-protein diet reduces the concentrating ability of the kidney by reducing the medullary gradient.

190. (D) Urea transport through the medullary collecting duct is enhanced by ADH.

191. (B) The urea clearance is higher at high urine flows, i. e., at lower urine to plasma creatinine ratios.

192. (E) Urate transport occurs mainly in the proximal segment and is carrier mediated.

193. (C) In one hospital, 19.5% of all hyperuricemias were caused by diuretics.

194. (A) Sulfinpyrazone is uricosuric.

195. (A) Uric acid is most highly concentrated in the deepest part of the medulla.

196. (C) Aspirin in high doses is uricosuric.

197. (B) Uric acid hypoexcretion occurs in lead poisoning; overproduction occurs in the other conditions.

198. (A) In the other conditions, uric acid levels may be disproportionately high.

199. (A) It is exceptional for gout to occur in sickle cell disease.

200. (D) Hypouricemia may occur in anaplastic carcinoma of the lung due to Fanconi's syndrome.

201. (B) Transmission is a sex-linked recessive gene.

202. (E) The syndrome occurs only in boys; development in the first 6 to 8 months of life is usually normal.

203. (D) In diabetes mellitus with glycosuria but without ketosis, hypouricemia may occur as a result of the inhibition of intratubular glucose on urate reabsorption.

204. (C) Salicylates in small doses suppress secretion; in large doses they suppress both the secretion and reabsorption of urate.

205. (B) Decreased extracellular volume increases proximal urate reabsorption.

206. (B) Beta-hydroxybutyric acid depresses tubular secretion of uric acid.

207. (C) The cause of the hyperuricemia in Down's syndrome is unknown.

208. (E) Xanthine oxidase abnormalities do not cause hyperuricemia.

209. (E) Glycosuria at low glucose levels occurs when the reabsorptive capacity of a segment of nephrons is exceeded.

210. (D) The carrier for glucose has not been isolated; phlorizin inhibits glucose reabsorption.

211. (A) Because of increased GFR, the filtered load may increase even if blood sugar falls.

212. (A) Aminoaciduria may be due to a direct effect on renal tubules, or an indirect result from changes in ion transport.

213. (A) Significant phosphaturia and bicarbonaturia suggest a proximal site of action.

214. (C) Initially, the poorly reabsorbed osmotic agent limits water reabsorption; hyperemia washes out the medullary gradient.

215. (C) Profound intracellular potassium depletion may cause entry of sodium into the cells, with a resultant decreased effect of plasma volume and hyponatremia.

216. (D) TcH_2O underestimates true water reabsorption because urine entering the collecting duct may be hypotonic, and because solutes are also reabsorbed from the collecting duct.

217. (A) Plasma renin levels increase with chronic diuretic use.

218. (D) Acetazolamide acts on the proximal tubule to produce phosphaturia.

219. (A) The kaliuretic effect is mainly distal; potassium repletion is more difficult than is usually assumed, because the supplements are excreted.

220. (B) Deafness has occurred with ethacrynic acid, and occasionally with furosemide, but not with the thiazide.

221. (D) Thiazides inhibit peripheral utilization of glucose.

222. (D) Furosemide acts slightly in the proximal tubule and inhibits reabsorption of sodium chloride and bicarbonate.

223. (A) Thiazides act at the cortical diluting site and impair dilution but not concentration ability.

224. (E) Thiazides act mainly on the distal convoluted tubule.

225. (B) Mersalyl acts in the diluting segment and inhibits active chloride reabsorption.

226. (E) Metabolic alkalosis is perpetuated by chloride deficiency, plasma volume contraction, and hyperaldosteronism; perpetuation by hypokalemia itself is rare.

227. (E) The increased urate reabsorption takes place in the proximal tubule.

228. (B) Respiratory compensation is by inhibition of the respiratory center; this can be harmful in chronic lung disease. Treatment is by chloride supplementation.

229. (D) Thiazides exert a therapeutically important effect in nephrogenic diabetes insipidus.

230. (E) Spironolactone produces minimal or no antidiuresis whereas the other diuretics may.

231. (E) Mercurials when given for short periods decrease K^+ excretion by blocking K+ secretion in the distal tubule and collecting duct not unlike amilonide and triamterene.

232. (A) Potassium-sparing diuretics are contraindicated in advanced renal failure because they can result in life-threatening hyperkalemia.

233. (E) A decrease in filtration fraction would probably cause antidiuresis.

234. (A) Furosemide is without effect on natriuresis when administered during maximal ethacrynic acid activity.

235. (A) Thiazides increase magnesium secretion.

236. (B) Ethacrynic acid has no proximal tubular effect.

237. (C) Organomercurials and furosemide have a high fractional sodium excretion.

238. (B) There is generally no rise in bicarbonate excretion.

239. (C) The major action of mercurials is on chloride reabsorption in the ascending loop.

240. (D) Furosemide abolishes the ability of the kidney to concentrate.

241. (C) The acute effect of furosemide may be venodilatation, thus allowing a pooling of blood and a decrease in the end-diastolic pressure.

242. (E) Bicarbonaturia occurs only acutely and is due to temporary carbonic anhydrase inhibition.

243. (A) Furosemide inhibits chloride transport in the ascending limb.

244. (D) Deafness and gastrointestinal bleeding occur mainly with ethacrynic acid.

245. (B) Furosemide has very feeble carbonic anhydrase

activity, but inhibits ATPase activity profoundly, and is not affected by changes in acid-base balance.

246. (C) Diuresis begins in 2 hours.

247. (D) Full natriuretic effect of spironolactone is usually delayed for a few days.

248. (D) Urinary concentrating ability is maintained.

2. CLINICAL EVALUATION OF RENAL FUNCTION

249. (D) Chyluria refers to lymph in the urine. The milky urine is due to triglycerides and a colloidal suspension of albumin, lecithin, cholestrin and soaps. Chyluria can be caused by lymphatic obstruction and filariasis.

250. (D) Eclampsia, fractures caused by accident, and carbon monoxide poisoning can cause loss of consciousness. They can also cause release of fat into the circulation and into the urine.

251. (E) Augmented sympathetic activity such as fright, pain, exercise, norepinephrine, and congestive heart failure will increase renal vascular resistance and reduce renal blood flow. GFR falls less because efferent arterioles are affected more by catecholamines.

252. (C) In nephrotic syndrome the low serum albumin will cause a fall in plasma oncotic pressure. Since GFR is governed by the difference between transcapillary hydrostatic pressure and colloid osmotic pressure, a fall in the latter will increase GFR.

253. (A) Hyperosmolar urine is found in volume depletion, acute glomerulonephritis, after infusion urography, and the hepatorenal syndrome.

254. (E) Albumin, a negatively charged ion, is normally repulsed by negatively charged glomerular glycoprotein. Loss of this glycoprotein may lead to increased filtration of albumin.

255. (A) Disease processes that disturb the function or structure of the medulla may be expected to produce early marked disproportionate impairment of concentrating ability.

256. (D) For each 30^oC above 16^oC, the specific gravity is 0.001 less than its true value.

257. (C) Selective proteinuria is characterized by the ability of the glomerulus to retain higher molecular weight proteins and permit filtration of lower molecular proteins such as albumin. This finding is typical of minimal change disease.

258. (B) Predominant tubular disease is associated with resistance to the action of vasopressin (Pitressin).

259. (C) In adrenal insufficiency diluting ability is grossly defective because of the lack of adrenal steroids.

260. (C) Creatinine excretion is 1 to 2 g/24 hr.

261. (C) Plasma osm = 2 x plasma (Na^+) + (glucose/18) + BUN/2.8.

262. (E) Patients with azotemia cannot concentrate maximally.

263. (A) Cadmium causes tubular damage and excretion of large amounts of $beta_2$-microglobulins.

264. (A) With moderate renal failure up to GFR of 10 ml/min, as the plasma creatinine rises, the rise in noncreatinine chromogen is much less and at the same time creatinine secretion increases, causing an overestimate of GFR by creatinine clearance method.

265. (B) Twenty-four-hour urine collections are notoriously inaccurate, the error frequently being inadequate urine collection. The error can be minimized by collection of two sequential 24-hour specimens.

266. (C) Urea is filtered, reabsorbed and secreted. Reabsorption is influenced by state of hydration. Urea production is also dependent on hepatic function and protein intake.

267. (A) Contrast media in a patient with diabetes mellitus can cause acute renal failure. The high osmolality is the result of glucose and some contrast material in the urine. Urine sodium is a more reliable indicator of acute renal failure in these patients.

268. (C) Inulin is freely filtered at the glomerulus and as it is neither reabsorbed nor secreted it accurately measures the GFR.

269. (E) In chronic pyelonephritis the kidneys are usually small.

270. (E) If appropriate end points are not achieved during water deprivation maximal urine-concentrating ability may not be achieved.

271. (A) Urine osmolality is more accurate than the rate or extent of urine excretion in assessing the maximum diluting capacity of the kidney.

272. (D) Maximal diluting and maximal concentrating ability of the kidney are impaired by diuretics.

273. (B) Even at low pH, the amount of acid excreted as free hydrogen is negligible and most hydrogen ion is excreted in the form of ammonium or titratable acids.

274. (D) Small contracted kidneys are difficult to biopsy but may be done in suitable subjects.

275. (E) Renal biopsy is unsafe on the right kidney since need for nephrectomy might result in uremia and it is not possible on the left. Renal vein renin activity may indicate a renovascular cause for the hypertension.

276. (D) Since the kidneys cannot be visualized and the patient is uremic, renal biopsy is contraindicated.

277. (A) Complement levels are normal in membranous glomerulonephritis.

278. (D) Marked pyuria is frequently seen in exudative glomerulonephritis.

279. (D) Reduced effective extracellular volume with reduced urinary loss of sodium is due to extrarenal sodium loss with avid sodium retention by the kidney.

280. (C) Hypoalbuminemia may result in decreased urinary protein excretion.

281. (D) The patient should be treated with antihypertensive

drugs, since renal biopsy is contraindicated while the blood pressure is high. Proteinuria is a feature of malignant hypertension, and may disappear with treatment.

282. (C) In acute oliguria, excess urinary sodium is due to acute renal failure or diuretics whereas with prerenal azotemia urinary sodium is low.

283. (A) Metabolic alkalosis with extrarenal loss of chloride such as from vomiting results in urine chloride of less than 10 mEq/L.

284. (E) The dip-stick, unlike the sulfosalicylic acid test, is not affected by turbidity, x-ray contrast media, or massive penicillin therapy.

285. (C) In prerenal azotemia, the urine to plasma urea concentration is usually greater than 10:1.

286. (B) Hyperuricemia, proteinuria, and old age are additional precipitating factors for reduction in renal function after IVP but hypouricemia is not.

3. HYPERTENSION

287. (D) Most major hypertension studies have used as diastolic blood pressure the point at which the sounds disappear, which can be significantly lower than the muffling point.

288. (E) If the arm is unsupported diastolic blood pressure may increase. In mild hypertensives diastolic pressure may increase in standing position. With rest, subsequent blood pressure readings may be lower than original readings.

289. (C) As many as 50% of patients do not adhere to prescribed therapy.

290. (B) The WHO criteria define normotension as systolic less than 140 mmHg and diastolic less than 90 mmHg.

291. (A) Borderline hypertensives usually have an increased cardiac output which may be from an overactive beta adrenergic nervous system. Blood volume is low and peripheral resistance is usually not elevated.

292. (A) Renovascular hypertension occurs in 2-5% of hypertensive populations studied.

293. (A) This range is recommended by the World Health Organization.

294. (E) All of the above have been associated with increases in blood pressure.

295. (C) Hypertensive blacks tend to have volume-dependent hypertension and a better response to diuretics than to beta blockers.

296. (A) There is evidence of increased sympathetic activity in essential hypertension, and increased hypertension in certain populations under social stresses.

297. (B) Pseudohypertension may occur in persons with stiff atherosclerotic vessels and sphygmomanometric readings may overestimate blood pressure in these elderly patients who may be particularly sensitive to medication.

298. (A) With the exception of renovascular hypertension, which occurs in 2-4% of the population, other forms of secondary hypertension rarely occur.

299. (D) Patients 25 or 30 years old should be investigated for secondary hypertension.

300. (D) If the rate of deflation of the cuff is done rapidly in a patient with a slow pulse, the true level of pressure may be missed.

301. (E) Evidence of sclerosis and narrowing may be found in both hypertension and arteriosclerosis.

302. (A) Despite current knowledge of the risk of hypertension, only a small percentage of patients have their blood pressure lowered properly.

303. (C) Most would obtain urinalysis, EKG, and blood chemistries initially.

304. (E) Renal fluid volume mechanisms are important only in long-term regulation.

305. (E) The essential hypertension pressure natriuresis curve is reset at the expense of a higher pressure. If this pressure is lowered by medication, sodium retention occurs.

306. (D) Most theories hold that in primary hypertension plasma volume is initially expanded. Most studies show that blood volumes are decreased when compared to normals, although they are too high for the degree of hypertension. Obese patients tend to be hypervolemic.

307. (A) In primary hypertension there is an increase in the filtration fraction with a normal GFR and decreased renal plasma flow.

308. (D) Efflux of Na is decreased in hypertensives.

309. (A) Natriuretic hormone is thought to be responsible for the exaggerated natriuresis in hypertensive individuals; it is highest in volume-expanded, low renin hypertensives: its source is unknown; its effect is caused by the inhibition of the Na-K-dependent ATPase which is responsible for the active extrusion of sodium and influx of potassium from cells. In renal tubules inhibition of this pump causes decreased reabsorption of sodium.

310. (E) Sodium in vessel wall is high in essential hypertension whereas it is normal in serum and urine.

311. (A) In essential hypertension blood flow is increased in muscle, decreased in the kidney, and normal in the liver, gut, and brain.

312. (A) There is evidence for higher intracellular calcium in essential hypertension, which may increase vascular tone and reactivity.

313. (D) Exaggerated rise in peripheral resistance during upright tilting reflects increased baroreceptor activity. This may be seen in borderline hypertension.

314. (C) Reduced renal blood flow may diminish uric acid excretion.

315. (C) Renin is a proteolytic hormone which acts on angiotensinogen to liberate angiotensin I and by itself has no pressor activity.

316. (E) Catecholamines decrease renal blood flow.

317. (B) PGI_2 escapes pulmonary degradation.

318. (A) The other conditions are associated with increased kallikrein excretion.

319. (A) Angiotensin infusion in a normal subject reduces glomerular filtration.

320. (C) The decaptide angiotensin I has no specific unique physiological action, but is cleaved in the lung by converting enzymes to yield the active octapeptide, angiotensin II.

321. (E) Angiotensin II stimulates aldosterone secretion.

322. (B) Its concentration is low after adrenalectomy, and high after nephrectomy.

323. (D) Indomethacin, a prostaglandin inhibitor, inhibits renin secretion; all the others stimulate renin secretion.

324. (D) Increased plasma potassium prevents renin secretion, all the others stimulate renin release.

325. (C) Angiotensin II has been shown to be a potent stimulator of thirst.

326. (E) Estrogen increases renin substrate which would cause an increase in plasma renin activity.

327. (C) Saralasin is a competitive agonist-antagonist to angiotensin II receptors.

328. (A) Estrogens increase renin substrate.

329. (B) Aldosterone is almost always increased in malignant hypertension, but may or may not be increased in the other condition.

330. (B) In Addison's disease the adrenals are primarily or secondarily affected so that aldosterone secretion is low.

331. (B) Intimal hyalinization is more severe with advancing age even in the absence of hypertension.

332. (A) Renin activity is determined by measuring angiotensin I production under controlled conditions.

333. (D) Proliferative endarteritis is characteristic of malignant nephrosclerosis.

334. (B) Collagen material external to Bowman's capsule suggests tubulointerstitial nephritis.

335. (A) The thrombus initiated by platelets later acquires the staining properties of fibrin.

336. (D) Arteriolosclerosis most extensively involves the kidneys, may occur with advancing age without hypertension, is almost always found with severe hypertension, and affects the afferent and efferent glomerular arterioles.

337. (B) In response to increased blood flow which delivers
338. (A) more nutrients to tissues, vessels in skeletal muscle
339. (A) constrict by autoregulatory mechanisms. Kidneys and brain maintain a constant flow through various perfusion pressures.

340. (A) PGF_2 is a vasoconstrictor whereas PGE_2 are
341. (C) vasodilatory. Glucagon has not been implicated in
342. (D) hypertension
343. (A)
344. (D)
345. (B)

346. (C) Liddle's syndrome is a renal tubular defect causing sodium retention and potassium excretion.

347. (D) Renin values are very low in Conn's syndrome.

348. (E) Azothioprine has not been associated with hypertension although it may cause liver toxicity.

349. (E) All of the choices may lead to encephalopathy.

350. (C) Cerebral hemorrhage in hypertension is due to Charcot-Bouchard aneurysms, usually in the internal capsule.

351. (C) The patient may show changes of malignant and benign nephrosclerosis, but not of renal vein thrombosis.

352. (C) Diffuse proliferative glomerulonephritis does not occur in primary malignant nephrosclerosis. Its presence signifies primary glomerular disease.

353. (D) Arthromatous emboli usually affect several organs.

354. (A) Cerebral tumors have been reported to clinically, but not biochemically, simulate pheochromocytoma.

355. (C) In toxemia there is a disproportionate reduction in urate clearance leading to hyperuricemia.

356. (D) Blood pressure usually decreases during the second trimester of a normal pregnancy, and should be considered severe.

357. (B) If used as the initial agent beta blockers may cause either a pressor response or pulmonary edema perhaps by removing the beta adrenergic drive to the heart associated with vasoconstriction mediated by unopposed alpha adrenergic stimulation

358. (A) Pheochromocytoma has been associated with neurocutaneous syndromes.

359. (D) These features are suggestive of catecholamine excess as seen in pheochromocytoma.

360. (E) The others listed will lower the VMA levels.

361. (A) In patients on maintenance hemodialysis hypertension is usually caused by increased intravascular volume and may be controlled by adequate ultrafiltration.

362. (B) In a young patient a careful urinary sediment examination should always be done to rule out glomerulonephritis.

363. (E) All of the choices should be considered in a young person with systolic hypertension.

364. (C) The above is suggestive of renal artery stenosis. Saralasin infusion test and intravenous urography have about equal false positive and false negative results and doing both would be unnecessary.

365. (A) In the one kidney model total body sodium is increased and plasma volume is expanded.

366. (E) High cardiac output states and rigid vessels all lead to systolic hypertension.

367. (D) Urine potassium usually exceeds 30 mEq/24 hr in a patient with primary aldosteronism.

368. (D) The other studies are only helpful in much larger tumors. The current limit for CT scan is 1 cm.

369. (C) The findings in this patient are suggestive of primary aldosteronism.

370. (D) Fibrinoid necrosis is the anatomical basis of malignant hypertension, and usually affects the media, sometimes the intima, and occasionally both.

371. (A) The patient may show changes of malignant and benign nephrosclerosis, but not of renal vein thrombosis or glomerulonephritis because of the mild proteinuria.

372. (D) Cerebral tumors may clinically, but not biochemically, simulate pheochromocytoma.

373. (D) Patients with renal and nonrenal causes of accelerated hypertension may have similar urinary findings, and renal function may be impaired in both.

374. (A) Dysplasias are more diffuse and result in the string of beads; poststenotic dilatation reflects the severity of the stenosis.

375. (E) All of the choices are associated with increased plasma volume.

376. (E) Fibromuscular dysplasia may occur at extrarenal sites and characteristically involves the distal sites of the renal arteries.

377. (B) Naloxone, a narcotic antagonist, may stimulate the sympathetic nervous system. Nose drops may contain sympathomimetics.

378. (B) Both minoxidil and hydralazine can cause palpitations and sodium retention as they are vasodilators.

379. (D) The other substances do not act on beta receptors.

380. (B) Prazosin is a postsynaptic alpha blocker and, as such, may be useful in pheochromocytoma. Starting with a 1 mg dose at bedtime has been suggested to prevent first-dose syncope.

381. (D) Captopril inhibits angiotensin-converting enzyme, thereby causing a reflex increase in plasma renin activity.

382. (C) Potassium-sparing diuretics should be avoided in patients with a tendency toward hyperkalemia.

383. (B) A common complication of hypokalemia from diuretics is digitalis intoxication.

384. (E) All are true.

385. (B) Both are central alpha adrenergic stimulants and are known to produce somnolence.

386. (D) Guanethidine can cause failure of ejaculation but usually not of erection.

387. (A) In patients not in heart failure cardiac output may be reduced and pulse may be slightly increased.

388. (D) Triamterene is a K+-sparing diuretic. Saralasin is an antagonist to angiotensin. Atenolol is water soluble.

389. (D) If a loading dose is not given, it may take several days for therapeutic levels to be reached.

390. (E) The stepped care program suggests that one dose of a drug should be used to the maximum that can be tolerated starting with a thiazide diuretic or a beta blocker. Minoxidil should be reserved as a step four drug.

391. (C) Nadolol has been shown to maintain renal blood flow while other beta blockers may decrease renal blood flow. Atenolol also has been shown not to decrease renal function.

392. (B) By interfering with renin secretion beta blockers can interfere with potassium metabolism. They also may inhibit release of insulin.

393. (A) Nitroprusside is a direct vasodilator. Captopril is an
394. (C) angiotensin-converting enzyme inhibitor. Methyldopa
395. (B) acts on the sympathetic nervous system. Phentolamine
396. (D) is a pure alpha-adrenergic blocker. Amiloride and
397. (E) chlorthalidone are both diuretics.
398. (D)

399. (A) The AV3V may be the source of natriuretic hormone.
400. (B) Lesions of the NTS cause hypertension in experimental
401. (B) animals which can be prevented by lesions in AV3V in certain animals.

402. (E) Clonidine may cause a rebound phenomenon. Sara-
403. (D) lasin may have stimulatory activity. Pindolol has
404. (C) intrinsic sympathomimetic activity. Propranolol may
405. (B) cause peripheral vasoconstriction. When given intra-
406. (A) venously guanethidine may release catecholamines.

407. (B) On intravenous urogram the kidneys may appear normal
408. (A) in chronic glomerulonephritis and nephrosclerosis. A
409. (C) disparity in size suggests renovascular disease, where-
410. (D) as distorted calyces suggest pyelonephritis. In nephrosclerosis protein excretion is usually less than 3.5 g/24 hr.

411. (C) The 11 hydroxylase deficiency is usually recognized
412. (C) in childhood; virilization is characteristic. The 17-
413. (D) hydroxylase deficiency produces hypogonadism. Both
414. (C) are treated with steroids, and both produce hyper-
415. (D) tension and hyperkalemia. The 3-beta-dehydrogenase
416. (A) deficiency is usually fatal in childhood and is asso-
417. (A) ciated with total absence of adrenal steroids.
418. (D)

419. (C) Both hyperplasia and adenoma result in hypokalemia
420. (B) and suppression of renin release. Plasma aldosterone
421. (B) falls in the upright position only in patients with aden-
422. (A) oma. Adrenal venous sampling differentiates the two
423. (A) conditions in 90% of cases.
424. (D)

4. DEVELOPMENTAL, VASCULAR, TUBULAR, AND NEOPLASTIC LESIONS

425. (A) There is patchy capillary wall thickening and sclerosis, but proliferative glomerulonephritis does not occur.

426. (B) Familial juvenile nephronophthisis is histologically identical with medullary cystic disease of the kidney.

427. (C) In medullary cystic disease inexorable progression to renal failure is the rule.

428. (D) Medullary sponge kidney is commonly diagnosed as an incidental finding on workup for urinary symptoms.

429. (E) Foam cells are found in many forms of renal disease but are most prevalent in hereditary nephritis, and have not been described in nephrosclerosis.

430. (E) Unilateral agenesis of the kidney is associated with arrested development of the Wolffian duct, resulting in nondevelopment of the rest of urinary tract on the affected side.

431. (E) Ureteral kinking and renal ischemia sometimes occur on standing but parenchymal damage does not occur.

432. (E) Renal vein thrombosis may be associated with glomerular damage and development of collateral renal veins.

433. (D) Hypernephroma with invasion of the veins, congestive heart failure, nephrotic syndrome, and often terminal complications of renal disease which has caused reduction in renal blood flow (e. g. , papillary necrosis) may be etiologic causes of renal vein thrombosis.

434. (C) Intense hemolysis occurs because of a substance present in donor plasma.

435. (B) This may be a response to the fibrin found near these cells.

436. (C) In one series 33% became hypertensive.

437. (D) Hyaline thrombi occur from intraluminal thrombosis associated with coagulopathies.

438. (D) Microangiopathic hemolytic anemia usually does not occur in Henoch-Schönlein purpura.

439. (C) The histologic appearance is most consistent with atheroembolic renal disease.

440. (E) Sex-linked dominant inheritance occurs in vitamin D-resistant rickets with females being heterozygous and males being homozygous.

441. (C) Primary RTA is probably transmitted as an autosomal dominant.

442. (A) Vitamin D-resistant rickets is transmitted as a sex-linked trait.

443. (E) Transport in the renal tubule and jejunum is defective in the other conditons.

444. (A) The protein in Fanconi's syndrome consists mainly of a mixture of globulins, and the proteinuria is much less than that seen in glomerular disease.

445. (D) There is only defective reabsorption of acidic and monaminomonocarboxylic amino acids.

446. (E) Arginine is found in cystinuria; the other four have a common transport mechanism that is absent in Hartnup's disease.

447. (E) The distal acidification system is intact in proximal renal tubular acidosis.

448. (A) If the filtered bicarbonate is lower than the tubular threshold, there will be complete bicarbonate reabsorption.

449. (B) Lowe's disease causes Fanconi's syndrome.

450. (1-D) Defective monoamino acid reabsorption leads to tryptophan deficiency
(2-B) Oculocerebrorenal syndrome
(3-A) The tubule is unresponsive to parathormone
(4-E) Nephrocalcinosis and calculi
(5-C) Defective glucose reabsorption with no symptoms

451. (C) Glycolipid accumulation in Fabry's disease is due to ceramide trihexosidase enzyme deficiency.

452. (B) Renal disease, however, is not present in all forms of familial hyperprolenemia.

453. (B) Children with tyrosinemia have nodular cirrhosis of the liver, and hepatoma is more common than in other types of hepatic cirrhosis.

454. (C) Pellagra caused by defective absorption of tryptophan from the jejunum is found in Hartnup's disease.

455. (E) It is inherited as a sex-linked recessive character. Renal function is normal except that the tubules are unresponsive to ADH, but the female heterozygote shows only diminished concentration ability.

456. (E) Urine persistently hypotonic to plasma and unresponsive to vasopressin may be encountered in diseases primarily damaging the tubules such as obstructive uropathy, chronic pyelonephritis, medullary cystic disease, amyloidosis, and nephrocalcinosis.

457. (B) Tubular epithelium gives rise to adenocarcinoma of the kidney.

458. (B) Metastases may regress after removal of the primary carcinoma.

5. PROTEINURIA, GLOMERULONEPHRITIS, AND THE NEPHROTIC SYNDROME

459. (C) Contrast media could also give a false positive test.

460. (A) Microscopical hematuria is usually not prominent in minimal change disease.

461. (D) Maltese crosses are actually fat bodies seen under phase contrast microscopy. They occur in the nephrotic syndrome.

462. (C) Most of the normal urinary protein is tubular in origin and are globulins.

463. (E) The paper strip test does not detect Bence Jones proteins.

464. (B) Tamm-Horsefall protein is excreted normally in the urine, and may be incorporated in hyaline casts. These dissolve in alkaline urine.

465. (D) Polycystic renal disease does not usually cause nephrotic proteinuria.

466. (E) None of these statements about renal vein thrombosis is correct.

467. (E) All of these conditions could cause renal vein thrombosis.

468. (C) The nephrotic syndrome by definition has to begin with urinary protein loss.

469. (D) All of these statements about the nephrotic syndrome are correct.

470. (C) The increased VLDL causes lactescanse of nephrotic serum. HDL and LDL are usually decreased with severe proteinuria. It has not been established that there is an accelerated rate of atherosclerosis in nephrotic patients.

471. (B) Serum 25-hydroxy-vitamin D is decreased in the nephrotic syndrome.

472. (C) Whereas IgM is decreased in the nephrotic syndrome IgG and IgA are decreased.

473. (A) The normal GBM usually excludes substances having a molecular weight more than 40,000 daltons.

474. (B) The absolute rate of albumin catabolism is probably unchanged or decreased whereas the fractional rate of catabolized albumin as a proportion of serum albumin is increased.

475. (B) Plasminogen actually increases in the nephrotic syndrome.

476. (C) The prognosis for renal function in orthostatic proteinuria is excellent.

477. (B) Quinidine has not been reported to cause the nephrotic syndrome.

478. (B) Polycystic renal disease does not usually cause nephrotic proteinuria.

479. (C) Soluble immune complexes usually occur in slight antigen excess.

480. (D) These substances all cleave C1.

481. (C) Aggregated IgA could activate an alternate pathway.

482. (C) The etiologic relationship to acute glomerulonephritis is uncertain.

483. (D) The pathogenetic significance of these findings is under study.

484. (E) The exact mechanisms remain unclear.

485. (D) The human glomerulus does have receptors for C3B.

486. (B) Serum C3 is normal in Berger's disease (IgA nephropathy).

487. (E) Acute nephritic syndrome is the most common presentation.

488. (C) The rate of relapse after a remission by prednisone is about 60%.

489. (C) There was a greater decrease in mortality after the introduction of penicillin than after prednisone.

490. (B) Lipoid nephrosis occurs at the time, or just shortly before, clinical Hodgkin's occurs.

491. (E) The cause of the relationship is uncertain, although believed to be immunologic.

492. (C) A plasma factor has been identified in the serum that would inhibit PHA-induced blastogenesis in lymphocytes.

493. (C) Proteinuria in focal segmental sclerosis is nonselective.

494. (D) Properdin levels are normal in lipoid nephrosis.

495. (D) Epithelial cell foot processes are not fused in benign nephrosclerosis. Fusion could be seen in any condition that gives rise to proteinuria.

496. (C) Hypertension is not usually a feature of lipoid nephrosis.

497. (C) About two-thirds of patients with lipoid nephrosis would have remission in 2 years without treatment.

498. (B) Infection remains the most common cause of death in lipoid nephrosis, but mortality is nowadays extremely rare.

499. (D) Segmental sclerosing lesions may be seen in repeat biopsies of long-standing lipoid nephrosis. This sclerosis has the same prognostic significance as the focal segmental sclerosis detected in early biopsies in the nephrotic syndrome.

500. (E) Focal and segmental sclerosis could be seen in a variety of glomerular diseases.

501. (C) Perhaps about 20% of cases of focal segmental sclerosis may respond to prednisone.

502. (E) Sclerosis may be a pathological response to any type of glomerular injury.

503. (D) Electro-dense deposits in membranous nephropathy could be subepithelial (epimembranous) or intramenbranous. Sometimes they could be identified in very early cases when light microscopy shows normal glomeruli. Before the days of fluorescent and electron microscopy, some of these cases must have been labelled as lipoid nephrosis.

504. (C) Sometimes the nephrotic syndrome remits if the neoplasia is entirely eradicated.

505. (E) A variety of solid tumors have been reported in membranous nephropathy.

506. (D) Penicillamine may induce a membranous lesion.

507. (E) Gross hematuria is not usually seen in membranous nephropathy; microhematuria is occasionally seen.

508. (D) Membranous glomerulonephritis does not present with gross hematuria, it is mostly associated with solid tumors, and usually progresses to chronic renal failure. Subendothelial electron-dense deposits are not usually seen in MGN.

509. (A) Although there may be remissions and exacerbations, edema is usual at onset.

510. (C) Nephrotic proteinuria is a very common presenting feature. Large subepithelial humps could be seen in secondary syphillis, bacterial endocarditis, MPGN (type III), Henoch-Schönlein purpura. They would be least likely to be encountered in focal segmental glomerular sclerosis.

511. (E) All of these infections, and many others, have been reported to produce acute glomerulonephritis.

512. (E) Subepithelial electron-dense humps could be seen in a variety of glomerular diseases as indicated above. The ASO titer usually rises after streptococcal pharyngitis whereas the anti-DNAase-B titer usually rises after streptococcal skin infections. The alternative and the classical complement pathways are probably utilized in acute post-streptococcal glomerulonephritis (APSGN).

513. (E) The whole glomerulus and all the glomeruli in the biopsy specimen are involved by exudative and proliferative changes.

514. (E) There is no conclusive evidence that APSGN patients with more than 50% crescents respond to this therapy.

515. (C) Acute porphyria may cause electrolyte disturbances.

516. (A) Hypertension is a common presenting feature in APSGN due to Na^+ retention.

517. (A) Severe oliguria is not a good prognostic sign.

518. (B) A diuretic is a good choice since the hypertension is mainly due to circulatory overload from salt retention.

519. (B) Mesangial hypercellularity can persist for several months or years after APSGN.

520. (D) Glomerular crescents are not common in MPGN.

521. (E) Mesangial interposition may be seen in all of these conditions.

522. (D) Serum C1q and C4 levels are often normal in type II MPGN (dense deposit disease).

523. (A) C3 cleaving factors may be found in the serum of patients with SLE, and trace amounts may be found in normal individuals.

524. (D) Abnormalities in the alternate complement pathway occur.

525. (B) Scleroderma has not been reported to cause MPGN; mild hypercellularity may occur.

526. (C) This therapy is not very effective when oliguria and severe renal failure have already occurred.

527. (E) Crescentic glomerulonephritis usually pursues a rapid course to renal shutdown, especially when more than 80% of glomeruli are involved by crescents.

528. (C) Oliguria is not usually a presenting feature.

529. (D) Lipoid nephrosis does not cause a rapidly progressive renal failure. Sometimes there is oliguria and azotemia resulting from severe hypoalbuminemia and decreased effective arterial volume. This usually reverses with remission of proteinuria.

530. (E) There may be a role for plasmaphoresis early in the disease.

531. (C) Spontaneous recovery is not frequent in anti-GBM antibody GN. The serum titer of anti-GBM antibody does not correlate with the severity and outcome of the disease.

532. (B) Gross hematuria has no prognostic significance.

533. (B) Occasionally nephrectomy is attempted in desperation and rarely helps.

534. (E) Pulmonary hemorrhage is not unique to Goodpasture's syndrome.

535. (A) Recurrent attacks of gross hematuria are most commonly seen.

536. (A) The nephrotic syndrome does not occur in more than 10% of cases.

537. (B) The most common lesion on light microscopy is a focal and segmental proliferative glomerulonephritis. Rapidly progressive GN with crescents is rare. Mesangial IgA fluorescence could be seen in other conditions (e. g. , Henoch-Schönlein purpura and lupus nephritis).

538. (B) Serum complements are normal.

539. (E) Amyloidosis has fibrillar material in the mesangium.

540. (C) Vascular inflammation is not seen in IgA nephropathy. In the other four the features mentioned are shared between IgA nephropathy and Henoch-Schönlein purpura.

541. (E) Dermal IgG would be more suggestive of lupus.

542. (D) Hematuria may occur in several hereditary glomerulopathies.

543. (D) Glomerular histology is normal.

544. (B) Focal segmental glomerulonephritis is not seen in the acute phase of poststreptococcal GN.

545. (E) The explanation for recurrent disease is not entirely understood.

546. (C) The unresponsiveness to steroid therapy makes this lesion unlikely. In the United States nowadays long-standing rheumatoid arthritis is probably the most common cause of secondary amyloidosis affecting the glomerulus.

547. (B) The International Study of Kidney Disease in Children (ISKDC) reported very long remissions of the nephrotic syndrome with cyclophosphamide.

548. (C) The figures are 73% at 5 years, and 46% at 10 years. Among the causes of the primary nephrotic syndrome MGN probably has the best prognosis after minimal change disease.

549. (C) Repeat biopsies in long-standing steroid-responsive minimal change disease may show focal segmental or focal global (the whole glomerulus) sclerosis. These changes do not seem to impart a negative prognostic significance.

550. (C) Attempts are being made to develop laboratory models
551. (A) of the various types of glomerular injury.
552. (D)
553. (B)
554. (C)

555. (C) Linear deposition is believed to represent reactivity to intrinsic basement membrane material and granular deposition to discrete foreign material trapped in the basement membrane.

556. (A)
557. (C)
558. (A)
559. (A)
560. (B)
561. (A)
562. (B)
563. (E)
564. (A)
565. (D)
566. (D)
567. (C)
568. (B)
569. (C)
570. (A)
571. (D)
572. (C)
573. (B)
574. (B)
575. (D)
576. (B)
577. (C)
578. (C)
579. (B)
580. (A)
581. (B)
582. (D)
583. (B)
584. (E)
585. (C)
586. (G)
587. (A)
588. (F)
589. (F)
590. (D)
591. (B)
592. (G)
593. (E)
594. (A)
595. (C)
596. (E)
597. (D)
598. (B)
599. (F)
600. (A)
601. (C)

6. URINARY TRACT INFECTION AND INTERSITITAL NEPHRITIS

602. (B) Staphylococcus aureus pyelonephritis is caused by hematogenous spread.

603. (D) Proteus accounts for 44% of UTI in boys compared to only 5% in girls.

604. (B) Perinephric abscess is caused by staph aureus in 14% of cases.

605. (B) Kidneys are quite resistant to hematogenous infection, unless there is obstruction to urine flow.

606. (C) Shorter urethra predisposes women to UTI. Besides sexual activity, personal hygiene and other factors influence the rate of UTI.

607. (B) VUR is about five times more common among males than females and tends to occur in families. The exact mode of inheritance is not known.

608. (D) Refluxing papillae are generally located in both polar regions. The scarring occurs in early infancy.

609. (A) Eighty percent of recurrences involve new bacteria; childhood bacteriuria predicts a relatively high-risk group of patients for recurrent UTI and renal scarring.

610. (C) Even though their long-term outlook is comparable to nonbacteriuric pregnant women, they should be adequately treated because they have higher incidence of acute pyelonephritis and perinatal mortality

611. (A) Absence of antibody-coating indicates a favorable response to treatment while a positive test indicates possibility of relapse. It is not a very sensitive test for localization of infection.

612. (C)
613. (B)
614. (E)
615. (A)
616. (D)

617. (C) Systemic amphotericin-B is highly toxic and is rarely indicated; however, local bladder irrigation with it is very effective.

618. (D) This change is most helpful in end-stage kidneys in trying to determine the underlying cause.

619. (D) Hyperchloremic acidosis as a result of impaired renal excretion of acid is more often a feature of chronic pyelonephritis than chronic glomerulonephritis since it represents tubular dysfunction.

620. (B) Sixty percent have Proteus organisms.

621. (C) Transitional cell carcinoma is a late manifestation.

622. (E) These patients frequently present with oliguric acute renal failure.

623. (C) Secondary syphilis causes glomerulonephritis, the others an interstitial nephritis.

624. (A) Ammonium chloride, being acid, may precipitate uric acid crystals since at a pH below 7 urate is present largely as the ionized and poorly soluble uric acid.

625. (C) The others usually show acute interstitial cell infiltration in the adjacent medulla.

626. (B) This causes modularity of the kidney surface due to cortical atrophy. The other changes are more typical of chronic nonobstructive pyelonephritis due to other causes.

627. (C) Sterile pyuria is suggestive of analgesic nephropathy.

628. (A) Balkan nephritis does not occur in persons under 20 years old. It occurs mainly in valleys and only after living in the area for 10 to 15 years.

629. (C) Penicillin, cephalothin, and sulfonamides can produce a hypersensitivity interstitial nephritis. Sulfonamide also causes intrarenal crystallization, gentamicin causes acute renal failure.

7. METABOLIC DISEASES AND NEPHROLITHIASIS

630. (E) Increased erythropoietin content of both plasma and tumor has been reported in renal carcinoma; in cyst fluid of patients with erythrocytosis associated with cerebellar hemangioblastoma; in plasma and tumor homogenates in a patient with hepatoma; and in cyst fluid and plasma in both solitary and multiple renal cysts.

631. (B) Chronic cadmium intoxication may occur from environmental pollution and has been described in Japan.

632. (E) Low-molecular weight protein (20,000 to 30,000) in the urine that precipitates with nitric acid is peculiar to cadmium nephropathy; porphyrinuria occurs in lead nephropathy.

633. (E) The symptoms suggest inorganic mercury poisoning; dimercaprol (BAL) is usually given first and dialysis is done shortly after to remove BAL mercury complexes since the patient is oliguric.

634. (B) Fenfluramine is a weak base so urinary acidification may be of theoretical value in the treatment of overdosage.

635. (C) This causes a low interstitial sodium concentration in the medulla and results in impaired water reabsorption from the collecting duct.

636. (A) The vacuoles appear foamy and can disappear with potassium supplementation.

637. (D) Diluting capability is usually well preserved in hypokalemic nephropathy even with severe impairment of concentrating ability.

638. (E) Multiple vacuoles in the tubular epithelium, mainly in the proximal convolutions, are suggestive of hypokalemic nephropathy. Low serum K of short duration may not show these changes.

639. (A) When potassium loss is an isolated defect, a hyperchloremic acidosis strongly suggests renal tubular acidosis as the cause.

640. (C) This is due to the concentrated acid urine which occurs in people living in the tropics.

641. (B) 25-hydroxycholecalciferol is converted to 1,25-dihydroxycholecalciferol in kidney.

642. (A) Subcutaneous deposits of calcium and shortening of metacarpal bones occur only in pseudohypoparathyroidism.

643. (C) Nephrocalcinosis is not found in Fanconi's syndrome despite increased calcium in the urine.

644. (E) About 60% of stones contain calcium oxalate with or without calcium phosphate.

645. (E) In most cases of renal-stone disease no consistent abnormality is found.

646. (A) The majority of kidney stones contain calcium in combination with oxalate or phosphate.

647. (A) Phosphaturia has not been demonstrated as a cause of stones, indeed orthophosphate is widely used in stone prevention.

648. (D) A high-phosphate diet will decrease calcium excretion in the urine.

649. (B) Thiazide diuretics decrease stone absorption by decreasing calcium loss in the urine and increasing urinary pyrophosphate excretion.

650. (C) This is probably the main mechanism and allows calcium to remain in the bone and not be released into serum.

651. (D) The medullary structures (loop of Henle and collecting duct) have a predilection for calcium deposition.

652. (B) This condition is a sex-linked dominant trait, is associated with hypophosphatemia and has normal tubular response to parathormone.

653. (D) Nephrolithiasis may occur in 50% of the patients.

654. (D) There is increased urinary hydrogen ion excretion and systemic alkalosis possibly due to increased carbonic anhydrase activity in the tubule in hypercalcemia due to conditions other than hyperparathyroidism.

655. (D) In multiple myeloma the hypercalcemia is due to demineralization of the skeleton.

656. (A) Increased gastrointestinal absorption of calcium plays only a secondary role.

657. (E) Alkaline urine does not prevent calcium phosphate stone formation; acidification reduces stone formation.

658. (A) Pure uric acid stones are radiolucent because they contain no calcium or sulfur.

659. (A) Ten percent of ethylene glycol is metabolized to oxalate. Ascorbic acid is also metabolized to oxalate. Crohn's disease and intestinal bypass produce hyperoxaluria probably by increasing oxalate absorption from the bowel.

660. (B) Pyridoxine deficiency causes hyperoxaluria and may be corrected by pyridoxine supplements.

661. (D) Magnesium ammonium phosphate stones are found in association with infection with urea-splitting organisms: however, occasionally prolonged excessive use of alkali will result in these stones.

662. (D) Cystine stone formation generally begins in childhood and is usually bilateral.

663. (B) Uric acid and xanthine stones are radiolucent.

664. (E) Existence of nephrocalcinosis and renal stones may result from all of the above conditions except cystinuria unless cystinuria is associated with recurrent urinary tract infection.

665. (A) The solubility of cystine requires a pH of 8 to prevent stone formation.

666. (C) The magnesium ammonium phosphate stone almost invariably contains calcium phosphate.

667. (A-3) Are usually associated with infection
(B-2) Causes mucosal abrasions that cause bleeding and result in a brownish coat
(C-4) Are usually multiple stones
(D-1) Are usually small

668. (C) Mixed calcium oxalate/calcium phosphate stones constitute approximately 37% of all stones. Calcium oxalate is more abundant than calcium phosphate in this mixed variety. Pure calcium oxalate (26%) stones are more common than pure calcium phosphate (71%) stones.

669. (A) Maximal rate of recurrence is in first 2 or 3 years; about 50% recur within first 5 years.

670. (B) Pregnancy and renal stones do not affect each other adversely, except for slightly increased rate of UTI.

671. (D) Uromucoids are unidentified substances with molecular weight of more than 12,000 daltons. They promote calcium phosphate crystallization and aggregation.

672. (A) Despite increased intestinal absorption of calcium and hypercalcemia, there is a negative calcium balance largely due to loss of bone mineral.

673. (C) At all levels of net calcium absorption urine calcium excretion is higher, causing negative calcium balance in more than 50% of patients.

674. (D) Renal hypercalciuria is not amenable to low calcium diet; negative calcium balance is aggravated and PTH increases.

675. (C) Primary defect is intestinal hyperabsorption of calcium, in turn causing PTH suppression and decreased tubular reabsorption of calcium.

676. (E)
677. (D)

678. (F)
679. (B)
680. (A)
681. (C)

682. (E) Only 39% of men and 22% of women with hyperuricosuria and calcareous renal stones have hyperuricemia.

683. (B) Most of the oxalate absorption occurs in colon, which is essentially defunct after ileostomy, and not available for oxalate absorption. In pancreatic insufficiency, jejunocolic bypass, and other forms of steotorrhoea, calcium in the gut is precipitated by free fatty acids and is not available for oxalate precipitation. Ethylene glycol and methoxyflurane cause oxalate overproduction.

684. (B) Allopurinol is indicated only if uric acid excretion is more than 1 g/day, or if stone dissolution is desired. Uric acid is less dissociable than urate at acid pH, hence uric acid stones are more common than urate stones. Hot climate causes dehydration, leading to highly concentrated urine with low pH, which promotes stone formation. Probenecid is a uricosuric agent and hence contraindicated.

685. (D) Urease splits urea into water, ammonia, and CO_2; NH_3 hydrolyses to form NH_4OH; and CO_2 hydrates to form H_2CO_3, which yields HCO_3 ions. At high pH, HCO3 loses a proton to form CO_3 and sets the stage for struvite stone formation.

686. (B) Unlike renal hypercalciuria, the intestinal absorption of calcium is not elevated; negative calcium balance occurs due to bone demineralization.

687. (E) Uretheral obstruction is most likely to result in urinary infection. Instrumentation may be a factor here.

688. (A) In acute tubular necrosis total anuria is possible but unusual, and would last only a short time.

689. (E) Acute obstruction behaves like renal artery stenosis by producing high urine osmolality and low urine Na. Obstruction increases DNA synthesis and cell division as compared to the control kidney.

690. (E) In patients with hydronephrosis the red cell count may

be elevated possibly due to increased erythropoietin production.

691. (E) All of the drugs listed may produce bladder atony giving rise to clinical features suggestive of obstruction.

692. (E) Methysergide produces retroperitoneal fibrosis; warfarin may obstruct the urethra by retroperitoneal hematoma or luminal hemorrhage. Sulfadiazine produces obstruction by precipitating in the tubules; and analgesic abuse may lead to papillary necrosis with the papillae subsequently obstructing the ureters.

693. (C) Temporal arteritis is not associated with retroperitoneal fibrosis.

694. (B) Retroperitoneal fibrosis may follow the use of methysergide which is used for the prevention of migraine.

695. (C) In neurogenic bladder a saccule may form at the vesicoureteral junction leading to reflux.

696. (E) The tendency to reflux is greatest with birth and usually subsides with maturity; many cases are probably asymptomatic.

697. (D) The macrolide group of drugs (erythromycin) readily enter the prostatic secretions as they are soluble in the extremely how pH of the prostate.

698. (B) Prostatic infection usually is due to one of the common urinary tract pathogens. Due to low pH in the prostate most antimicrobials are ineffective.

699. (E) In partial ureteral obstruction, the urine volume may be normal, or even increased.

700. (C) In acute obstruction there is decreased filtration per nephron; in chronic obstruction there is an increase in GFR per nephron similar to chronic nonobstructive renal disease.

701. (B) There is no impairment of sodium reabsorption in the ascending limb of loop of Henle as evidenced by the preserved capacity to dilute the urine.

702. (C) The reason for this abnormality in obstructive nephropathy is unknown but it possibly is due to back pressure on the tubular cells.

703. (B) Postobstructive diuresis produces a large daily excretion of Na along with the other abnormalities described.

704. (E) Pneumaturia, though rare without a vesical fistula, sometimes occurs in diabetics especially with E. coli cystitis.

705. (D) Although milky urine may be found in lipiduria and pyuria, a milky appearance that varies with posture may suggest chyluria since it is produced by obstruction of lymph flow.

706. (D) Though all the components mentioned are present in chyluria the major component is triglycerides.

8. RENAL INVOLVEMENT IN SYSTEMIC DISEASE

707. (C) Glomerular filtration is elevated in early diabetic nephropathy.

708. (C) Both afferent and efferent glomerular arterioles are involved by diabetes.

709. (D) The linear pattern found in some diabetic kidneys reflects nonspecific basement membrane alterations and does not imply an immunologic mechanism.

710. (B) Arteriolosclerosis, not arteritis, is seen in diabetic nephropathy.

711. (B) Uncontrolled hypertension correlates best with the rate of progression of diabetic nephropathy.

712. (B) Hypertension is usually associated with nephrotic syndrome in diabetics.

713. (E) Nitrofurantoin may cause diffuse lung disease. The others may induce SLE.

714. (A) There is a poor correlation between the initial antinuclear antibody titer and the presence of active lupus nephritis.

715. (B) Hematoxylin bodies — amorphous ill-defined glomerular masses — are almost specific for lupus nephritis.

716. (C) Heavy proteinuria alone is not necessarily a sign of active lupus nephritis.

717. (C) Diffuse proliferative lupus nephritis has the worst prognosis, having only a 25% 5-year survival rate.

718. (C) The presence of peritubular and interstitial immune deposits would generally distinguish interstitial nephritis from the other conditions.

719. (D) Low-dose steroid therapy is often sufficient to control segmental lupus nephritis.

720. (E) About 30-50% of patients have a major flare in disease activity within 8 weeks after delivery. Because of this the dose of prednisone should be increased during that period.

721. (C) The incidence of renal manifestation in procainamide lupus is very low.

722. (D) Most affected patients are slow acetylators of hydralazine.

723. (B) Patients with mixed-connective tissue disease tend to have a very high titer of antibody to a saline-extractable ribonuclear protein antigen.

724. (D) A higher incidence of SLE has been reported with DRW_2 and DRW_3, also with B_7 and B_8 haplotypes.

725. (E) Over 90% of patients with untreated SLE have antibodies to double-stranded DNA.

726. (C) Glomerular microthrombi without necrosis have been observed in association with a circulating anticoagulant.

727. (B) Hemoptysis is not a characteristic feature of scleroderma.

728. (C) Pulmonary hemorrhage may be associated with a variety of renal diseases. Of these, Goodpasture's syndrome is characterized by a linear immunofluorescent pattern.

729. (D) The effectiveness of current regimens has largely eliminated the need for bilateral nephrectomy.

730. (A) Heavy protein loss rarely has time to occur because progression of renal disease is so rapid.

731. (C) The classical renal outcome is severe hypertension with renal shutdown.

732. (A) Serum complement levels in scleroderma are normal.

733. (D) Recovery from renal failure has been reported and contraindicates early nephrectomy.

734. (B) The nephrotic syndrome in endocarditis has been described but is unusual.

735. (E) Patients may develop nephrogenic diabetes insipidus from amyloid deposition around the collecting ducts.

736. (C) Hypertension is usually absent, even with advanced renal failure, although recent studies have suggested that in well-nourished patients mild to moderate hypertension may be present.

737. (E) The nephrotic syndrome is uncommon in periarteritis nodosa; the other features are commonly encountered.

738. (C) A telescoped urinary sediment, containing broad renal failure casts as well as evidence of active disease, may be seen.

739. (C) In polyarteritis nodosa hypertension is common and may be severe or malignant.

740. (D) Rapidly progressive glomerulonephritis with crescents and fibrinoid necrosis may occur in microscopic polyarteritis nodosa.

741. (A) Fibrinoid necrosis is characteristically seen in the glomerulus and in the arcuate and interlobar arteries.

742. (C) Striking diffuse deposition of IgA in the mesangium is characteristic of Henoch-Schönlein syndrome.

743. (C) Although there are features suggestive of allergin or

or immunologic factors, the serum complement component values are usually within normal limits.

744. (E) The mesangial location, the granular nature of the immune deposits, and the presence of IgA with chiefly the late-acting complement components including properdin suggest an immune-complex disease with activation of the alternate complement pathway.

745. (C) In adolescents, membranous lupus may precede all other clinical and laboratory evidence of SLE, and is frequently characterized by the presence of mesangial deposits.

746. (A) In contrast to the focal nature of the glomerular lesions by light microscopy, one of the striking features is the diffuse presence in the glomeruli of granular deposits of IgA, C3, and properdin.

747. (E) The prognosis has been considerably improved by treatment with cyclophosphamide.

748. (E) Cimetidine may cause an interstitial nephritis with eosinophils in the infiltrate.

749. (B) Renal failure from papillary necrosis is extremely unusual.

750. (C) Such filling defects have been mistaken for neoplasms or calculi, and have led to unnecessary nephrectomy.

751. (C) A nephrotic syndrome with fusion of foot processes only has been described with nonsteroidal antiinflammatory drugs. Gold and penicillamine may cause membranous nephropathy.

752. (D) Renal function generally remains normal during the course of gold nephropathy.

753. (D) When an osmotic diuretic is ineffective in acute hyperuricemic nephropathy immediate dialysis should be considered for removal of uric acid and treatment of uremia.

754. (A) The renal lesion is not associated with any clinical manifestations other than mild proteinuria.

755. (C) Colchicine is of possible value only in the amyloid associated with periodic mediterranean fever.

756. (C) Renal amyloidosis is quite uncommon.

757. (A) Alpha and beta globulins do not produce renal disease in myeloma.

758. (A) Renal concentrating defect is the result of tubular damage by Bence Jones protein and also hypercalcemia.

759. (D) Hyaline thrombi constitute the hallmark of thrombotic thrombocytopenic purpura.

760. (D) Hypertension is common and may become severe as the disease progresses.

761. (D) The alkaline phosphatase is usually normal in multiple myeloma.

762. (C) In multiple myeloma hypertension and persistent hematuria are rare.

763. (C) Mesangial IgA deposits are characteristic of Berger's disease. The other conditions have been associated with membranous glomerulopathy.

764. (A) Carcinoma of the stomach has been associated with membranous glomerulopathy, the others with the mesangiocapillary (membranoproliferative) variety.

765. (A) Sarcoidosis has been associated with other forms of glomerulonephritis, but not with minimal change.

766. (C) Endocarditis is the most likely diagnosis, and focal necrotizing glomerular lesions are typical.

767. (E) Concentrating ability is usually well maintained; diluting ability is lost.

768. (C) There is poor renal perfusion in Laennec cirrhosis because of shunting of blood to other areas.

769. (C) This constellation of clinical features is most suggestive of amyloidosis.

9. RENAL FAILURE

770. (E) The muscle destruction is associated with myoglobinuria and rapid increases in phosphate, urate, creatinine, and muscle enzyme levels.

771. (B) Rapid reduction of the serum potassium level during hemodialysis may cause arrythmias in digitalized patients.

772. (E) Thrombosis of the large renal arteries is seldom seen.

773. (E) Corticosteroids do not prevent renal necrosis; they may actually produce it after bacterial toxins are injected.

774. (C) Of the cases of cortical necrosis, 50% result from premature separation of the placenta.

775. (E) Large renal arteries remain open in cortical necrosis; the afferent and efferent arterioles may be occluded.

776. (D) Up to 300 ml/hr/m^2 may be lost between the fifth and tenth days after a burn.

777. (A) Five-tenths percent silver nitrate solution is hypotonic; electrolytes seep into the dressings, and hyponatremia ensues if electrolyte replacement is inadequate.

778. (B) Mafenide (Sulfamylon) inhibits carbonic anhydrase and reduces titratable acidity in the urine.

779. (D) This solution is closest to an ultrafiltrate of plasma.

780. (E) Muscle destruction leads to the liberation of myoglobin, but more than half of the patients also have severe dehydration. The renal failure associated with gentamicin is not associated with rhabdomyolysis.

781. (C) Carbon tetrachloride classically causes severe acute hepatic damage and rather insidious onset of acute renal failure.

782. (D) With modern dialytic therapy this remains the major complication.

783. (B) In acute tubular necrosis, the U/P creatinine is less than 14:1 .

784. (A) Although early lots of vancomycin occasionally caused renal injury, nephrotoxicity has not been observed with currently used preparations.

785. (D) Severe gastritis and upper GI bleeding are associated. with accidental or suicidal ingestion of mercuric chloride.

786. (C) Oxalate crystals are seen in ethylene glycol poisoning but not with bichloride of mercury.

787. (1-D) Ethylene glycol causes acute renal failure with cal-
(2-B) cium oxalate deposition; the other agents tend to
(3-A) cause more chronic processes.
(4-C)
(5-E)

788. (E) Ethylene glycol is rapidly metabolized to oxalic acid, which precipitates in renal tubules causing acute renal failure and other effects.

789. (B) Sulfonamide or uric acid crystalization, blood clots, hematomas, and retroperitoneal fibrosis may cause obstructive uropathy; indomethacin produces none of these.

790. (B) Usually all nephrons are affected to a similar degree.

791. (C) Tetracyclines have an antianabolic effect by preventing protein synthesis from amino acids thus worsening the azotemia by the direct production of urea. This effect is minimal with the use of doxycycline.

792. (B) In the presence of acute renal failure the urinary sodium concentration is usually high because the damaged tubules cannot reabsorb sodium.

793. (C) In acute renal failure (acute tubular necrosis) some residual urine output is usually maintained; with gentamicin high-output renal failure is often seen.

794. (E) Although urine alkalinization and mannitol have been shown to modify the amphotericin B toxicity in animals, it has not been helpful in humans.

795. (E) The basal requirement is about 400 ml; to this must be added various measured losses.

796. (D) The emergency treatment of hyperkalemia is glucose, insulin, and sodium bicarbonate to drive potassium into the cells pending more definitive therapy.

797. (B) Sodium reabsorption by the proximal tubules increases as a result of decreased effective plasma volume.

798. (C) Cortical blood flow decreases from 80 to 10% while corticomedullary flow increases from 14 to 80% of the total renal blood flow respectively.

799. (A) Chloramphenicol has not been associated with the production of acute renal failure; 90% of the drug is metabolized by the liver.

800. (A) Alkalinization may prevent the cast deposition in the tubules. Diuretics alkalinize the urine.

801. (E) In ethylene glycol nephropathy the tubules are usually filled with calcium oxalate crystals which are birefringent on polarized light.

802. (E) LeVeen shunt, in which peritoneal fluid is directed to jugular vein, is associated with dramatic increase in urine volume and sodium excretion.

803. (C) The toxicity of carbon tetrachloride is potentiated by alcohol because the former is soluble in alcohol and this increases its absorption.

804. (D) Severe gastrointestinal bleeding is classically seen in mercuric chloride poisoning because of this agent's corrosive effect on the gastrointestinal mucosa.

805. (C) Renal medullary necrosis usually occurs in elderly diabetics with preexisting urinary tract infection and overwhelming renal infection.

806. (D) Acute tubular necrosis is characterized by inability of the tubule to reabsorb filtered sodium. The renal failure index and urine sodium concentration are less sensitive measures of this than the fractional excretion of sodium.

807. (D) The urine osmolality remains low.

808. (D) In addition to insensible loss, each degree increase in temperature (F) above normal requires an additional 7%/hr of body weight of fluid.

809. (D) Experimental studies suggest that acute uremia inhibits the proliferation of fibroblasts and the formation of granulation tissue.

810. (B) Complete anuria for more than 48 hours should suggest ureteral obstruction, bilateral renal artery obstruction, renal cortical necrosis, or acute glomerulonephritis.

811. (E) In the hepatorenal syndrome sodium reabsorption is usually intense, and the urine sodium is low.

812. (E) Exhausted deionizers can cause water to leach copper from tubing and cause acute copper poisoning with hemolysis.

813. (B) In acute tubular necrosis from 5 to 10% of filtered Na is excreted.

814. (C) Though several conditions in myelomatosis may cause acute renal failure, tubular blockage by Bence Jones protein is by far the most common.

815. (D) Fractional excretion of sodium is calculated by the formula:

$$\frac{\text{urine sodium}}{\text{serum sodium}} \times \frac{\text{serum creatinine}}{\text{urine creatinine}} \times 100$$

816. (D) In hyperkalemia calcium infusion is the most rapidly effective method for treating cardiac toxicity.

817. (B) A concentrating defect persists for many months when other renal functions have recovered.

818. (D) The trade-off hypothesis is that as a result of certain efforts by the body to correct a metabolic abnormality seen in chronic renal failure, other undesirable bodily effects occur. Parathormone may stimulate the kidney to excrete phosphate but at the same time it damages bone.

819. (B) Considering the maximal concentrating ability of the kidney, this is the smallest amount of urine that is necessary for maintaining homeostasis.

820. (B) With progressive renal failure the interval of administration for procainamide should gradually be lengthened to 6, 8, or 12 hours.

821. (E) Although in normal subjects the renin angiotensin system is most important, in the anephric state potassium is most important.

822. (C) The metabolic clearance rate of aldosterone in chronic renal failure is high which is due to possible hyperdynamic circulation and increased hepatic degradation.

823. (D) The urine in advanced renal failure is isotonic, so approximately 300 mOsm are excreted in each liter.

824. (A) Uric acid clearance tends to fall less than creatinine clearance as a result of decreased reabsorption and increased secretion.

825. (D) The urine volume in renal failure is primarily limited by the low glomerular filtration rate.

826. (A) The occurrence of hypertension accelerates the progression of renal damage and atherosclerosis, and increases the rate of progression of uremia.

827. (D) Magnesium intoxication causes weakness, hyporeflexia, and quadriplegia. The symptoms may be reversed by calcium administration.

828. (D) Water moves into the brain and the brain pH may become lower than before dialysis.

829. (A) With high flux rates the delivery of acetate to the patient may exceed his capacity to metabolize it, resulting in inadequate correction of acidosis and possible shunting of acetate into alternative metabolic pathways.

830. (B) Papilledema is a complication of hypertension.

831. (A) Hemiparesis is not regarded as a manifestation of the disequilbrium syndrome.

832. (C) Since the filtered load of sodium is decreased in chronic renal disease, each surviving nephron is in a state of diuresis and excretes a greater percent of the filtered sodium.

833. (C) With increasing degrees of acidosis in chronic renal failure there is a greater degree of impairment of ammonium excretion than titratable acid.

834. (E) Hepatitis is a complication of dialysis, not of uremia.

835. (A) Free water clearance when expressed per 100 ml of GFR in chronic renal disease is frequently within the normal range.

836. (E) Acidosis, anemia, polyuria, and osteodystrophy, as well as recurrent infections, and protein malnutrition interfere with the normal growth of the uremic child; neuropathy, however, would generally be a late phenomenon.

837. (D) Rapid and profound hypotension during dialysis ultrafiltration is a likely sign of tamponade.

838. (A) Hyponatremia and not hypernatremia can exaggerate the electrocardiographic abnormalities of hyperkalemia.

839. (A) Uremic pericarditis is almost always bloody, usually painful, and may often persist in the dialysis patient for quite some time.

840. (B) Systemic heparinization may cause pericardial hemorrhage and is to be avoided if possible in uremia.

841. (B) Pericarditis is more common in patients who are under dialysis and if felt to be due to accumulation of unidentified substance which is dialyzable. This type of pericarditis seems to be different from pericarditis in a patient with chronic renal failure who has never been on dialysis.

842. (A) The pulse rate usually increases.

843. (C) The incidence and severity of neuropathy depend largely on the timeliness of dialysis.

844. (C) Wristdrop is characteristic of lead poisoning, and would be most unusual in the peripheral neuropathy of renal failure.

845. (E) Definite cause for decreasing incidence of neuropathy is not well understood. The noticeable difference in dialysis treatment may be responsible for this. Vitamin replacement does not have any significant role.

846. (D) Nitrofurantoin may cause polyneuropathy in uremic patients indistinguishable from uremic polyneuropathy. Penicillin and dilantin in high doses may also cause the same.

847. (A) Asymptomatic uremic neuropathy occurs in at least 50% of all patients with end-stage renal failure or who are on maintenance hemodialysis.

848. (D) Uremic neuropathy begins in the lower extremities.

849. (D) Severe peripheral neuropathy may not respond to dialysis but may improve within 6 months after transplantation.

850. (E) Increasing the calcium concentration in the dialysate may cause hypercalcemia and metastatic calcification in this patient; parathyroidectomy is the preferred treatment here.

851. (C) Dialysate calcium levels should be maintained at about 7 mg/100 ml.

852. (C) The common predisposing factor toward metastatic calcification is elevation of the circulating CaxP product resulting from high phosphate in CRF. This is accentuated in an alkaline environment.

853. (C) In chronic renal failure, the conversion of 25-OH vit D_3 to 1-25 $(OH)_2$ vit D_3 in the kidney is decreased or absent; however, 25 OH vit D_3 may increase calcium absorption. The other listed agents have a more direct effect on bone disease.

854. (D) Osteosclerosis producing horizontal bands of increased bone density of vertebrae gives the characteristic Rugger Jersey spine.

855. (D) In dialysis patients T_4 conversion to T_3 is impaired. T3 levels are low, T_4 normal or low, and TSH levels normal.

856. (C) There is a paradoxical response of growth hormone in patients with CRF. After administration of glucose instead of decreasing, growth hormone increases. Growth hormone is usually elevated.

857. (B) Hemodialysis produces no detectable alternations of the concentration of gastrin from the normal physiology.

858. (C) All of the gastrointestinal symptoms improve with dialysis except the incidence of peptic ulcer-related disease.

859. (C) With progressive destruction of nephrons, maintenance of external balance for salt requires an increased fractional salt excretion as GFR decreases.

860. (D) Dialysis dementia develops in patients on chronic hemodialysis. It is characterized by dysparaxia, myoclonus, seizure, and is not responsive to therapy.

861. (C) Other than cardiovascular complications, cerebrovascular accident is the next most common cause of mortality in long-term hemodialysis patients. The other listed conditions are less frequent causes and can frequently be managed with medical therapy.

862. (E) The main defect is hypertriglyceridemia, possibly from defective peripheral very low-density lipoprotein catabolism. High-density lipoproteins are reduced, and fatty acids rise only after dialysis, because of heparin.

863. (A) Testosterone levels are reduced in dialysis patients.

864. (A) Parathormone levels have been correlated with the blood urea.

865. (D) Dialysis dementia does not improve with dialysis and in fact is occasionally worsened.

866. (A) In uremia, the degradation of insulin in the kidney is impaired.

867. (D) Insulin antagonism is probably the main cause of the carbohydrate intolerance in uremia.

868. (B) Chloramphenicol is rapidly inactivated in the liver, where it is conjugated to the monoglucuronide. Additional doses should be administered after dialysis.

869. (E) A number of drugs such as chloramphenicol, isoniazid, phenylbutazone, and phenothiazines interfere with phenytoin metabolism, thus increasing blood levels and half-lives.

870. (B) A serum ferritin value in the low-normal range is at present the most convenient indicator of the necessity for iron replacement in dialysis patients.

871. (C) Malignant nephrosclerosis may cause severe proteinuria. In other listed conditions there is insignificant or absent proteinuria.

872. (B) Each functioning glomerulus filters an increased sodium load and hence fractional sodium excretion increases.

873. (C) The most striking abnormality in acid-based regulation in renal failure is impaired ammonia output by the tubule.

874. (A) Bicarbonate diffuses slowly in CSF which therefore remains acidotic in spite of the serum pH correction; this continues to stimulate respiration.

875. (D) The bone carbonate acts as a buffer by exchanging hydrogen ion for calcium.

876. (D) Fluid overload is one of the factors responsible for accelerated hypertension in patients with chronic renal failure on maintenance hemodialysis. The process of ultrafiltration removes water thus correcting the blood volume and blood pressure and should be the first line of therapy.

877. (D) Accumulation of cephalosporin and penicillin may

cause seizure in patients with renal failure. Discontinuation of the particular drug reverses symptoms. Accumulation occurs because the drugs are excreted by the kidney.

878. (D) Only ethambutol is excreted by the kidney and its dose should be reduced to 5 mg/kg/day. Phenytoin catabolism is slowed down by isoniazid.

879. (D) Increased delivery of sodium to distal exchange sites will result in increased sodium reabsorption at distal sites in the presence of impermeant anions which raise the transtubular potential difference, with resultant increase in potassium and hydrogen secretion.

880. (E) Hyperkalemia is associated with type IV renal tubular acidosis.

881. (B) Rapid correction of extracellular acidosis by fast hemodialysis or infusion of $NaHCO_3$ is followed by respiratory alkalosis because there is a lag in the correction of cerebrospinal acidosis.

882. (D) Transfusions may occasionally be indicated, but it is generally not possible or desirable to maintain a normal hematocrit.

883. (D) It is possible that extrarenal erythropoetin secretion may occur.

884. (C) Erythrocytosis may occur during transplant rejection possibly as a result of reduced nephron perfusion and increased erythropoietin secretion.

885. (D) Release of platelet factor III improves with dialysis, thus improving bleeding diathesis which is one of uremic complications.

886. (C) A dialyzable uremic toxin is felt to be the cause of abnormal platelet functions which include both defective release of factor 3 and platelet aggregation inhibition. Hemodialysis, peritoneal dialysis, and transplant correct these abnormalities.

887. (D) Even when hematocrit is 25-30 the presence of angina pectoris is an indication for blood transfusion in patients with chronic renal failure.

888. (C) Plasma fibrinogen is usually raised and fibrinolytic activity is usually depressed, but they return to normal following adequate dialysis.

889. (A) Cortical necrosis does not reduce peritoneal clearances. In the other conditions hemodialysis may be indicated if optimal clearances are needed.

890. (D) A specific defect in the activity of platelet factor 3 has been observed in uremia.

891. (E) The clearance of larger molecules such as inulin is increased.

892. (D) Dialysance is useful in evaluating dialyzer efficiency; clearance is useful in evaluating how much solute is removed from the patient

893. (E) Removal of water depends largely on hydrostatic pressure.

894. (A) The dose of 1 mg/kg may be given at intervals equal to eight times the serum creatinine; or the dose divided by the serum creatinine can be given at 8 hourly intervals; or the 8 hourly dose should be reduced to 0.2 to 0.5 mg/kg depending on how low the clearance is.

895. (A) Kanamycin is removed by peritoneal dialysis.

896. (E) The substances listed are in descending order of clearance; the uric acid clearance is somewhat lower than that of creatinine.

897. (B) Hyperglycemia draws water out of cells and establishes a gradient which favors diffusion of sodium from the peritoneal fluid into the extracellular space. Thus water is removed in excess of the isotonic proportion of sodium. As glucose is metabolized the water returns into the cells and hypernatremia persists.

898. (E) This technique facilitates fluid removal. It may help with control of ascites and hypertension.

899. (E) When renal function is normal more than two-thirds of an administered dose of carbenicillin is recovered in the urine within 6 hours. The recommended dose in severe renal failure is 2 g every 12 hours.

900. (C) Aluminum hydroxide is regularly prescribed and is a frequent cause of constipation.

901. (E) Fluid films and flow patterns largely determine the solute transport in dialyzers.

902. (C) The cause of gynecomastia is unknown; a similar phenomenon has been described in malnourished inmates of prison camps who were refed.

903. (A) Zirconium phosphate absorbs the ammonia produced by the action of urease on urea.

904. (E) Urea is removed mainly by diffusion, not osmosis.

905. (B) Copper intoxication has been reported to cause acute hemolysis.

906. (C) Constrictive pericarditis with maintenance dialysis was thought to be rare, but in recent years has been described more frequently.

907. (A) These are symptoms of formaldehyde infusion.

908. (D) The respiratory center is still stimulated because of lag in correcting the CSF acidosis, and thus there is hyperventilation.

909. (A) Dialysance takes into account the blood flow rate, the arterial and venous concentrations, and the concentration of solute in the dialysate, but not the dialysate flow rate.

10. PREGNANCY AND THE KIDNEY

910. (B) Plasma volume increases by about 50%.

911. (B) Cardiac output increases by 30-40%.

912. (B) Average creatinine level is 0.46 ± 0.06 mg/100 ml.

913. (B) The GFR is increased 40-50% with pregnancy resulting in a low BUN.

914. (C) Progesterone induces a natriuresis by inhibiting the sodium-retaining action of aldosterone.

915. (E) Chloride rises to compensate for the respiratory alkalosis of pregnancy; generally the concentrations of the others fall during pregnancy.

916. (C) Aldosterone is secreted in very large amounts in pregnancy.

917. (D) Standing causes pressure on the vena cava by the uterus.

918. (E) While routine use of diuretics is not recommended, their occasional use has not been shown to be harmful.

919. (C) Oxytocin has an antidiuretic effect.

920. (D) Some 20% of untreated bacteriuric women may develop acute pyelonephritis.

921. (D) Although the differential diagnosis may be difficult, chronic glomerulonephritis is the most likely diagnosis.

922. (D) Glomerular endothelial swelling is the characteristic renal lesion.

923. (B) A short, fat body build predisposes a woman to preeclampsia.

924. (B) Preeclampsia has not been reported in coarctation of the aorta.

925. (C) Bed rest is more effective in mobilizing fluid than a low-salt diet or diuretics which may cause volume contraction and aggravate circulatory insufficiency.

926. (E) Complement and immunoglobulins have not been demonstrated in the kidney in preeclampsia.

927. (A) The mechanism is unknown but cannot be reversed by aldosterone antagonists.

928. (D) In essential hypertension, unlike preeclampsia, the serum uric acid is normal and the urate to inulin clearance ratio is not decreased.

929. (C) Serum lactate is elevated and thus blocks secretion of uric acid.

930. (B) Hydralazine is widely used, but so are methyldopa and, increasingly, propranolol.

931. (E) Deposits in glomeruli consist of fibrin.

932. (B) Pregnancy and delivery are normal in the majority of women, although a few have toxemia.

933. (A) Improvement of toxemia is related to delivery of the placenta, as there is no improvement with retention of the dead fetus in utero.

934. (A) The blood pressure frequently falls during the second trimester.

935. (E) The estrogens secreted by the placenta normally elevate all these substances. In toxemia probably because of placental ischemia, these values are reduced from the normally elevated levels.

936. (C) Uric acid clearance in pregnancy is increased, perhaps because of extracellular volume expansion.

11. IMMUNOLOGY AND TRANSPLANTATION

937. (A) Antibody to basement membrane antigen is developed in a different animal species, and this antibody is injected into the animal being studied.

938. (E) This is an immune-complex type of nephritis.

939. (D) There are dense deposits on the outer side of the basement membrane.

940. (E) Experimental manipulations to study immunologic pathways have shown that neither complement nor polymorphonuclear leukocytes are essential in acute serum sickness although they appear to be involved in chronic ongoing immune-complex nephritis.

941. (D) Large complexes formed in slight antigen excess are the most potent and bind the most complement.

942. (C) Chronic serum sickness nephritis is a chronic membranoproliferative lesion induced by repeated foreign protein injections to maintain only slight antigen excess.

943. (B) With moderate excess of antigen most of the complexes are insoluble, whereas either extreme lack or excess of antigen or antibody produces fewer insoluble complexes.

944. (E) Immune-complex-induced glomerulonephritis constitutes more than 80% of all cases. Many tubulointerstitial diseases (e.g., methicillin nephritis) have been shown to be induced by immune-complex mechanisms.

945. (E) Antigens usually contain multiple potential binding sites, and most antibodies have two potential binding sites.

946. (E) Antigen-antibody complexes are found by immunofluorescence in the other conditions.

947. (E) Diffuse glomerulonephritis occurs when antigen is present in high concentration relative to antibody, allowing the formation of small (class) immune complexes.

948. (A) IgA and IgM immunofluorescence only appears in later stages of the disease.

949. (A) There is little evidence to suggest that PMNL are the primary initiating factor for tissue damage in immune-complex disease, and depletion of circulating PMNL does not affect the glomerular lesions in foreign protein nephritis.

950. (A) Patient A probably has lipoid nephrosis. The other patients may have immune-deposit disease from malaria, secondary syphilis, Staphylococcus albus bacteremia, and endocarditis respectively.

951. (B) Alport's syndrome is not an immunologic disease.

952. (D) Fibrinogen and IgA are the most common substances found by immunofluorescent staining in this condition.

953. (E) The membrane attack mechanism is activated via C5 to C9.

954. (E) Complement activation stimulates phagocytosis.

955. (E) C4b, 2a, 3b form C5 convertase which splits C5 into two fragments.

956. (C) There is no correlation between the clinical severity of the disease and immunofluorescence for C3.

957. (C) Linear GBM fluorescence for IgG has been reported in SLE, focal segmental sclerosis, diabetes mellitus, normal autopsied kidney, in 10% of normal kidney biopsies, and in kidney grafts after perfusion.

958. (E) Since finely granular deposits may mimic the linear pattern of antibasement membrane glomerulonephritis, the diagnosis should be confirmed by electron microscopy, serology, and by the presence of antibasement antibodies especially after nephrectomy.

959. (A) The decline of anti-GBM antibodies is usually complete in 6 months following nephrectomy and the serum assay should be determined before transplantation.

960. (B) Immunofluorescence particularly for IgG and C3 is present in the finely granular complexes of membranous glomerulopathy and absent in lipoid nephrosis; this is particularly important when light microscopic differentiation of the two lesions is not possible.

961. (C) In membranoproliferative disease the deposits are mainly in the subendothelial region whereas in poststreptococcal glomerulonephritis they are in the transmembranous and subepithelial region.

962. (B) By immunofluorescent study it has been shown that benign essential hematuria is usually associated with IgA deposition in the mesangium.

963. (C) Anti-RNA and anti-ENA antibodies are rarely connected with lupus nephritis while anti-DNA antibodies appear to play the greatest role in producing the renal changes.

964. (E) Cytotoxic antibodies may be induced by blood transfusions and pregnancy, and recently have been described in a variety of infections and autoimmune states.

965. (E) Cytotoxic antibodies are more common in this condition due to the combined effects of pregnancy and blood transfusion, even if separated in time.

966. (E) There is no specific immunofluorescent pattern in rapidly progressive glomerulonephritis, and numerous patterns have been described.

967. (A) This is usually found in lupus patients with mild proteinuria and normal light microscopy findings.

968. (B) The gamma globulin causing immunofluorescence in Goodpasture's syndrome is IgG.

969. (A) Most series report only capillary wall staining to fibrinogen.

970. (E) All of the systems play a part.

971. (A) The cells appear near the endothelial cells of capillaries and venules within a few hours of transplantation.

972. (B) Circulating antibodies are produced in the spleen and regional lymph nodes by lymphocytes activated into plasma cells.

973. (A) Iodohippurate (Hippuran) clearance falls before any other functional evidence of rejection appears.

974. (E) All but antinuclear antigens have been shown to play a role in the rejection process.

975. (A) The mixed lymphocyte culture tests showed the highest percent of reliability in predicting graft survival but it cannot be performed in cadaver transplantation because time is needed to do this test; of the other tests, the lymphotoxicity test is more reliable.

976. (A) There is enhanced rosette formation in response to recipient mononuclear cells.

977. (E) The antibody binds to HLA antigen on the vascular endothelium.

978. (C) Donors and recipients should conform in blood groups, otherwise hyperacute rejection will probably occur.

979. (A) Hypertension is often a sign of acute or chronic rejection and if it does not respond to antirejection therapy it should be investigated by biopsy and angiography, etc.

980. (D) Hyperacute rejection is resistant to all forms of therapy and can be prevented only by careful pretransplant evaluation.

981. (B) The high parathormone levels in the presence of normal vitamin D metabolism will increase calcium reabsorption and phosphate excretion, and the high parathormone levels may promote bone resorption and cause hypercalcemia.

982. (E) There is inhibition of monocyte but not granulocyte chemotaxis.

983. (E) Pancreatitis may occur in 5-15% of the patients and may be caused by steroids, high PTH levels, surgical trauma, infection, or even immunologic disease, and carries a grave prognosis.

984. (A) No recurrence has been reported in medullary cystic disease.

985. (A) Isografts and syngeneic grafts are between two totally identical individuals; xenograft and heterografts are transplants across species; an allograft is one within a species but not identical.

986. (D) Both siblings are a one haplotype match. In order to determine the best donor an MLC test should be done which may indicate the degree of compatibility at the LD locus and improve the chances of success.

987. (A) Assuming both donor 1 and 2 have equal HLA-A and HLA-B compatibility, donor 1 is more suitable since his lymphocytes cause the least stimulation of the recipient's lymphocytes. The mithromycin-treated cells in this test serve as antigenic stimulation to the nontreated cells in the mixed lymphocyte culture.

988. (A) The crossmatch is performed to determine if the recipient is already sensitized to the cells of the donor since such sensitization would lead to rejection of the donor's organ.

989. (A, C) Pulmonary infection is a frequent cause of death in immunosuppressed patients with chronic lung disease; oxalosis seems to recur within a few months in transplanted kidneys. In patients with Fabry's disease, transplant of a kidney containing galactosidase may actually improve the patient's symptoms; cysteine in transplanted kidneys of patients with cysteinosis has not been a serious problem.

990. (A) The histologic picture suggests cytoxic antibody reaction to vascular epithelium similar to what causes a hyperacute rejection; since it is occurring several weeks after transplant and not in the first few hours it is called accelerated.

991. (C) There is frequent fulminant recurrence of oxalosis; in Alport's syndrome careful screening of living donors should be done; patients with posterior valves may require an ileal conduit.

992. (D) Skin cancers appear mainly in sun-exposed regions and are usually multiple and the outlook is good.

993. (B) Skin and lip cancers are most common followed by non-Hodgkin's lymphomas and carcinomas of the uterine cervix. Other tumors are seen less frequently in transplant patients than in the general population.

994. (C) The cause of this condition is uncertain; although immunologic factors are suspected, the histologic evidence is usually minimal.

995. (C) Only a viable kidney will take up hyppurate. The other tests might be misleading; both conditions cause elevation of BUN and creatinine and the urine findings may be misleading if the native kidneys are still elaborating urine.

996. (B) Preformed donor-specific antibodies coat the vessels as soon as blood flow is established and this stimulates platelet aggregation and fibrinogen activation resulting in vascular thrombosis.

997. (B) The infiltrate is usually sparse; there is mainly interstitial edema. The other cells listed are found in acute cellular rejection.

998. (E) Although azothioprine is metabolized by the liver and can cause liver toxicity, myelosuppression is the most common manifestation of toxicity. With impaired renal function, the dose of azothioprine may need to be reduced.

999. (B) Cyclosporin is only mildly toxic to hematopoetic cells other than the lymphoid series.

1000. (B) The lesion consists of mild mesangeal proliferation and increase in matrix, occasional reduplication of the basement membrane, and subendothelial deposits of IgM, IgG, C_1 and C_3.

1001. (E) Over 90% of recipients shed CMV in the first several months after transplant. Leukopenia, hepatitis pneumonia, and GI bleeding can be clinical manifestations.

REFERENCES

1. Wyngaarden, J. B. and Smith, L. H., eds., Cecil Textbook of Medicine, 16th ed., 1982. W. B. Saunders Co., Philadelphia Pa.

2. Petersdorf, R. G., et al., eds., Harrison's Principles of Internal Medicine, 10th ed. 1983. McGraw-Hill Book Co., New York.

3. Heptinstall, R. H., Pathology of the Kidney, 3rd ed., 1983. Little, Brown and Co., Boston.

4. Laragh, J., ed., Hypertension Manual, 1974. Yorke Medical Books, New York.

5. Maxwell, M. H. and Kleen, C. R., Clinical Disorders of Fluid and Electrolyte Metabolism, 3rd ed., 1980. McGraw-Hill Book Co., New York.

6. Berliner, R. W. and Orloff, J., eds., Handbook of Physiology, Sec. 8-Renal Physiology, 1973. Williams & Wilkins, Baltimore.

7. Earley, L. E., Gottschalk, C. W., Strauss, M. B. and Welt, L. G., Diseases of the Kidney, 3rd ed., 1979. Little, Brown and Co., Boston.

8. Schrier, R. W., ed., Renal and Electrolyte Disorders, 2nd ed., 1980. Little, Brown and Co., Boston.

9. Kaplan, N., Clinical Hypertension, 3rd ed., 1982. Williams and Wilkins, Baltimore.

10. Brenner, B. H. and Rector, F. C., eds., The Kidney, 2nd ed., 1981. W. B. Saunders Co., Philadelphia.

11. Gonic, H. C., ed., Current Nephrology, (Vol. 1) 1977. Pinecliff Medical Publishing Company, Pacific Palisades, Calif.

12. Breener, B. M. and Stein, J. H. , eds. , Contemporary Issues in Nephrology (Vols. 1-10) 1978-1983. Churchill Livingstone, New York.

13. Black, D. , and Jones, M. F. , Renal Disease, 4th ed. , 1979. Blackwell Scientific Publications, Oxford, London.

14. Hamburger, J. et al. , eds. , Advances in Nephrology, (Vol. 1-4) 1971. Year Book Medical Publishers, Chicago.